CONTENTS

Introduction   v

Instructor's Guide

Chapter 1	Health Care of the Elderly: An Overview	1
Chapter 2	Characteristics of Nursing Homes	6
Chapter 3	Assessment of the Nursing Home Resident	9
Chapter 4	Common Health Problems of Residents in Nursing Homes	12
Chapter 5	Medication Use in the Elderly	17
Chapter 6	Acute Illnesses and Health Emergencies	20
Chapter 7	Documentation Requirements in the Nursing Home	23
Chapter 8	Health Protection and Promotion in the Nursing Home	26
Chapter 9	Subacute Care	29
Chapter 10	Philosophy and Structure of the Nursing Home	32
Chapter 11	Organization and Function of the Nursing Department	35
Chapter 12	Role of the Charge Nurse	38
Chapter 13	The Survey Process	41
Chapter 14	The Quality Improvement Process	44
Chapter 15	Legal and Ethical Issues in the Long Term Care Setting	48

Testbank

	Questions	Answers/Rationales
Chapter 1	51	105
Chapter 2	53	106
Chapter 3	57	108
Chapter 4	62	112
Chapter 5	72	118
Chapter 6	76	121

	Questions	Answers/Rationales
Chapter 7	80	123
Chapter 8	82	125
Chapter 9	84	126
Chapter 10	87	127
Chapter 11	90	129
Chapter 12	93	130
Chapter 13	97	133
Chapter 14	100	134
Chapter 15	102	135

INTRODUCTION

I believe that nursing is an interpersonal activity. That is, nursing takes place between two or more people and has health and help as central elements. Learners in nursing need to acquire skill in critical thinking and content knowledge as well as experience working with groups. Further, learning is best accomplished with active participation by learners. Educational materials should be presented in ways that facilitate learners' ability to master necessary interpersonal skills as well as factual content.

Critical thinking has been variously defined. All definitions indicate that critical thinking allows the learner to demonstrate a variety of thinking skills. Among those skills are the ability to define problems and set goals by clustering data; to gather information through use of all senses and by formulation of appropriate questions; to retrieve information from various sources; to organize information by comparing, grouping, and sequencing; to analyze information by examining parts and relationships, finding main ideas, and identifying errors; to produce new information by elaborating and inferring what may be true; to summarize by combining information into a succinct statement; and to evaluate information by using a standard for measurement. The ability to think critically requires extensive practice and learning materials that do not give the learner an immediate "right" answer.

Working with groups requires that learners mutually determine goals, plan appropriate agendas; accomplish goals within time constraints and summarize progress; give and receive ideas by setting an open atmosphere and by building on ideas; encourage and appreciate others by seeking the participation of all group members, processing the feelings/attitudes of all members, and valuing individual differences; and finally, work within the group by creating and assigning group roles and responsibilities. Many learners have little experience with the interpersonal skills needed to work effectively within a group. Indeed, one leading educator estimated that as many as 80 percent of new graduates terminated from their first job were discharged because they could not work with others rather than because they had poor knowledge of their job.

Cooperative learning, as a teaching strategy, has demonstrated that learners are able to improve performance with critical thinking and interpersonal skills. Cooperative learning has several crucial elements that distinguish this teaching strategy from group work. Those critical elements are positive interdependence, individual accountability, attention to interpersonal skills, and task structuring. Positive interdependence is perhaps best characterized by Ben Franklin's famous, "We must all hang together or we will most certainly all hang separately." Individual accountability means that each learner is evaluated based upon his or her own efforts. The main complaint that learners have about" group work" is that others may benefit unduly, or they themselves may be penalized, from the work effort of the group. Iinterpersonal skills or social skills such as tolerant listening, constructive criticism, or seeking clarification need to be modeled and practiced at all levels of education. The final element, task structuring, means that the teacher must structure group work so that no learner can easily complete the task alone.

Forming groups should be done with some care. It is not a good idea to permit learners to form their own groups. We prefer to work with our friends, and we try to avoid the challenges of working productively with those we view as different from ourselves. Teacher-formed groups permit learners to encounter classmates in different forums. Groups should be formed with an eye to diversity, high scorers and low scorers, introverts and extroverts, experienced and inexperienced. Ideally, groups should contain no more than four members. Cooperative learning takes place in face-to-face dialogue. Thus, larger groups cut the available interaction time for the group members. Group members should be given clear-cut tasks such as recording group decisions, timekeeping, to ensure that the task is completed in the allotted time, encouraging the participation of all group members, and giving positive feedback.

Despite teachers' best efforts and hard work, some combinations of learners are tormenting to all concerned. Teachers need to make provisions for varying group membership, such as rotating one member, on a routine basis. The rotation accomplishes at least two positive outcomes. One, learners encounter a wider number of their classmates. Two, knowing that someone they have difficulty working with is not on permanent assignment improves outlook toward group activities. Groups need time to adjust to one another in order to be most productive. Rotation should be done after 10 to 12 class hours if possible.

Electronic information sources are essential for learners to use, in addition to traditional print material. However, learners commonly complain that they do not know how to evaluate sources or materials that are available. Instructors as well as learners find that "surfing the Net" can consume a great amount of time. I have tried to include in each chapter instructors' resources that give actual Internet addresses to appropriate sources of information. Each address should be rechecked for accuracy before learners are given assignments. I strongly suggest that instructors give learners a brief introduction to the Internet and a brief written guide of search strategies before they give assignments using electronic resources.

Some curricula will use *Introduction to Long Term Care* as the primary text for instruction in the nursing care of the older adult. Other curricula may use the text as part of an orientation to the role of the nurse in a long term care setting, with more attention focused on managing care effectively. As a consequence, courses will cover differing content in varying depth. The instructor's guide for each chapter includes an outline of chapter contents, a description of the chapter contents with suggestions for using content for shorter and for longer courses, a list of Internet resources, and critical thinking exercises including group Internet or other assignments, discussion questions, and a case study. Instructions are given on how to format the Internet assignments and case studies as group assignments. Instructors may find that the exercises are appropriate for individual written assignments. The content description suggests chapter material that should be emphasized if a course requires completion in a shorter period. For longer courses, additional chapter material that should be emphasized is identified.

Elaine Bishop Kennedy, EdD, RN

CHAPTER 1

HEALTH CARE OF THE ELDERLY: AN OVERVIEW

OUTLINE

Demographics of Aging
Health Status of the Elderly
Health Care Settings for Elders

ORGANIZATION AND CONTENT

Chapter 1 briefly describes the population that learners will encounter. The chapter also introduces the political, social, and economic contexts for the health care of elderly people.

For shorter courses, because Chapters 1 and 2 describe the social underpinnings for nursing homes, they can be assigned together to form an introduction to the nursing home environment.

For longer courses, students can be directed to investigate community resources, both health care and community-based programs, that exist to meet the needs of elderly people. Students can also be given one or two Values Clarification exercises to help them determine their own attitudes toward aging and the elderly population. The first Values Clarification Exercise can set the stage for fact-finding.

INTERNET RESOURCES (BE SURE TO CHECK EACH ADDRESS.)

U.S. Administration on Aging (AOA)
Aging-related libraries and databases
http://www.aoa.dhhs.gov
This source provides links to academic libraries, statistical research centers, and state information sources.

http://www.ageinfo.org/data.html
This source provides a link to a set of statistical profiles on older Americans.

National Bureau of Economic Research (NBER)

NBER Center for Aging Research
http://nber.harvard.edu/aging.html
The NBER is one of nine centers for research on the demography and economics of aging funded by the National Institute on Aging.

CRITICAL THINKING EXERCISES

Group Assignment

Ask groups of learners to go on-line to find information on these demographic characteristics of people over age 65: age, gender, marital status, and socioeconomic status. Each group could be assigned to a different subgroup or different cultural or ethnic group of elders.

Discussion Items

Ask learners to:
- Identify elders who are at greatest risk for poor health and explain why.
- Predict the health behaviors of an elder with dizziness and blurred vision who has great trust in the health care system.
- Predict the health behaviors of an elder with frequent shortness of breath while walking who has little trust in the health care system.
- Explain why the population of elderly is growing so rapidly.
- Compare and contrast health care settings for the elderly.

Case Study

Present the following case study to the class. After giving learners the information, break them into groups for discussion. Ask one person to be the recorder, one to be the timekeeper, one to present the group's decisions to the class, and one to ensure that all members contribute to the discussion.

> Juan Hernandez is a 75-year-old Hispanic-speaking man who lives at home with his wife. Mr. Hernandez operated his own lawn maintenance service for many years and still enjoys working daily outdoors. Recently he has noted that he is easily fatigued after a little physical activity. At a cookout, Mr. Hernandez tells his neighbor, who is a nurse, "I'm running out of steam too easily these days. I just don't seem to have any 'get-up and go' left." Mr. Hernandez' neighbor suggests that he make an appointment to be seen by his health care provider as soon as possible.

Group One

- What knowledge about health status and the elderly, in general, would be helpful for the nurse to know?

Group Two
- Does Mr. Hernandez' culture have any impact upon his predicted life expectancy? Upon the likelihood of his being admitted to a nursing home?

Group Three
- What factors may influence Mr. Hernandez with regard to making and keeping an appointment with his health care provider?

Group Four
- Mr. Hernandez is most likely to use which health care setting? Is it likely that he will be in a health maintenance organization?

VALUES CLARIFICATION EXERCISES

Values Clarification Exercise 1

Put the following 10 items on an overhead transparency, or photocopy and hand them to learners. Ask learners to determine whether the statement is TRUE or FALSE. (All answers are false.) Be sure to discuss the rationales offered for any true responses in a nonjudgmental manner.

FACT OR FICTION?

1. All the needs of the elderly can be met by the services of a nursing home.

2. All older people are neglected or ignored by family.

3. Most elderly people feel that it is their children's responsibility to care for them in old age.

4. Grandparenting is universally enjoyed.

5. As people grow older, they grow more alike.

6. Elderly people, as individuals or as workers, are less creative, productive, and efficient than other people.

7. Older people tend to be inflexible.

8. The performance of elderly people on intelligence tests is lower than that of younger adults.

9. Most older people are lonely and isolated.

10. Old age is sexless.

Values Clarification Exercise 2

Give learners the following poem and allow them a few minutes to read it. Ask them to discuss the assumed age and gender of the writer, the writer's feelings about his or her life, and the overall message of the poem.

I WOULD PICK MORE DAISIES

If I had my life to live over, I'd dare to make more mistakes next time.

I'd relax. I'd limber up. I would be sillier than I've been this trip.

I would take fewer things seriously, take more chances, take more trips.

I'd climb more mountains, and swim more rivers.

I would eat more ice cream and less beans.

I would, perhaps, have more actual troubles, but I'd have fewer imaginary ones.

You see, I'm one of those people who lived seriously, sanely, hour after hour, day after day.

Oh, I've had my moments, and if I had it to do over again, I'd have more of them.

In fact, I'd try to have nothing else, just moments, one after another—instead of living so many years ahead of each day.

I've been one of those persons who never goes anywhere without a thermometer, hot water bottle, a rain coat, and a parachute.

If I had it to do over again, I would travel lighter this trip.

If I had my life to live over, I would start going barefoot earlier in the spring and stay that way later in the fall.

I would go to more dances, I would rider more merry-go-rounds.

I would pick more daisies.

> Anonymous

CHAPTER 2

CHARACTERISTICS OF NURSING HOMES

OUTLINE

History of Nursing Homes
Nature of Nursing Homes and Their Residents
Finance and Reimbursement Issues in Nursing Homes
State and Federal Regulations Governing Nursing Home Care
Accreditation of Nursing Homes
The Nursing Home as an Organization
Implications for Long Term Care Nursing

ORGANIZATION AND CONTENT

Chapter 2 details the history of nursing home development and the political decisions that facilitated the growth of the nursing home industry. Various types of nursing homes are described by their ownership and their populations. Nursing home residents are described in general. The dynamics of the transition process from living in the community to residence in a nursing home is described. Governmental regulation and regulatory agencies are identified.

For shorter courses, Chapter 2 can be combined with Chapter 1 as a brief overview of the political, social, and economic framework for nursing homes. It is most important to discuss family dynamics and relocation syndrome in the transition to nursing home care.

For longer courses, a more in-depth discussion about the types of nursing homes and the regulations governing the operation of long term care facilities should be undertaken.

INTERNET RESOURCES (BE SURE TO CHECK ADDRESSES.)

Joint Commission on Accreditation of Healthcare Organizations (JCAHO)
http://www.jcaho.org
JCAHO is a private, nonprofit organization dedicated to improving quality of care in a variety of health care settings, including long term care.

Health Care Financing Administration (HCFA)
http://www.hcfa.gov
HCFA is a federal agency within the Department of Health and Human Services. It was created in 1977 to administer the Medicare and Medicaid programs.

CRITICAL THINKING EXERCISES

Group Assignment

Ask learners to:

- Provide a short description of the mission and history of the JCAHO and HCFA using JCAHO and HCFA information, such as a printout.
- Differentiate between Title XVII (Medicare) and Title XXIX (Medicaid)
- using information from HCFA, such as a printout.
- Develop a list of information sources in the area to which elders can be
- referred for answers to their questions about Medicare and Medicaid.

Discussion Items

Ask learners to:

- Describe how the long term care needs of people under age 65 differ from those of elders.
- Differentiate between extended care facilities and subacute care units.
- Discuss the economic and social factors that lead to short-stay residents and long-term residents.
- Develop a profile for elderly residents at greatest risk for relocation syndrome.

Case Study

Present the following case study to the class. After giving learners the information, break them into groups for discussion. Ask one person to the recorder, one to be the timekeeper, one to present the group's decisions to the class, and one to ensure that all members contribute to the discussion.

> Mr. Sean McGregor, a mildly confused 93-year-old man, was admitted to the nursing home this afternoon. His wife died 4 months ago. His two daughters, aged 75 and 73, have been trying to convince him to stop living alone and move "where someone can look out for you." Mr.

McGregor has resisted making the commitment but agreed to "look over" a placement. His daughters made arrangements for admission and packed his clothes in a suitcase. While Mr. McGregor is on a tour of the facility, they leave the suitcase and drive off. The next day Mr. McGregor becomes very loud and agitated.

Group One
- What factors place Mr. McGregor at risk for relocation syndrome?

Group Two
- What negative health outcomes might be predicted for this resident?

Group Three
- What behaviors should the nurse anticipate from Mr. McGregor?
- How should the nurse respond to Mr. McGregor's statement "I can't find my clothes! Someone's taken my clothes" when his clothing is in his closet?

Group Four
- What measures could have been taken to prevent relocation syndrome for this resident?

CHAPTER 3

ASSESSMENT OF THE NURSING HOME RESIDENT

OUTLINE

Physiologic Changes Associated with Aging
Laboratory Test Values Affected by Aging
Psychosocial Changes Associated with Aging
Assessment of Residents in Young and Middle Adulthood
Assessment of the Newly Admitted Nursing Home Resident
Focused Assessments
Transfers to Other Health Care Settings

ORGANIZATION AND CONTENT

Chapter 3 details the numerous physical changes, including significant laboratory test results, that are affected by aging. The major psychosocial impacts of aging are also described.

For shorter courses, learners should be directed to review their notes on human growth and development as they relate to the developmental tasks of the age 65 and over population. Learners should also be directed to review the developmental tasks of the young and middle adult. The elements of assessment for newly admitted residents to a nursing home are covered in detail. It is most important to cover age-related physical and psychosocial changes.

For longer courses, the assessment of the newly admitted resident should be highlighted, as well as the tools for documentation that the nurse will encounter. A discussion of the responsibility of the RN versus the LPN/LVN for the initial nursing assessment should also be included.

INTERNET RESOURCES (BE SURE TO CHECK ADDRESSES.)

University of Florida Medical School
http://www.med.ufl/medinfo/geri/topics.html
Contains all the elements to be included in a thorough medical evaluation of an elderly resident. Directions to other resources are included in the text.

Sample Minimum Data Set (MDS)/Resident Assessment Protocol (RAP)/Care Plan: http://www.pca-computran.com/~lifesty/mdscare.htm
Contains examples of an MDS, a RAP, and a care plan derived from the information on the other two documents.

CRITICAL THINKING EXERCISES

Group Assignment

Ask learners to:

- Select one major body system, such as the cardiovascular system, and develop a list of age-related changes for both physical findings and common laboratory tests.
- Select one major psychosocial change associated with aging, and develop an assessment guide to document resident findings for that area.

Discussion Items

Ask learners to:

- Identify eight normal aging changes in body systems.
- Discuss whether retirement is a positive or negative life event.
- Discuss how developmental tasks may be interrupted by admission to a nursing home for adults of all ages.
- Describe how daily assessment of residents may differ from daily assessments of clients in acute care.

Case Study

Present the following case study to the class. After giving students the information, break them into groups for discussion. Ask one person to be the recorder, one to be the time keeper, one to present the group's decisions to the class, and one to ensure that all members contribute to the discussion.

> Mrs. Inez Connor, widowed and aged 71, has been diagnosed with Alzheimer's disease for 3 years. Her general health has been good. Her son Jim reports that now even the simplest task, such as showering, requires careful supervision. Jim and his two sisters are unable to maintain their jobs and young families and provide Mrs. Connor with the 24-hour supervision she requires. With deep reluctance, Mrs. Connor and her family agree to admission to a nursing home.

- ***Group One***
  Which assessments, both physical and mental, would be important for the nurse to make during the initial assessment?
- ***Group Two***
  In which laboratory tests would the nurse expect to see values greater than the ranges considered normal for young or middle adults? Why?
- ***Group Three***
  What areas on the RAPs would the nurse expect to address for Mrs. Connor? (Direct students to Appendix B in the textbook for sample RAPs.)
- ***Group Four***
  Who is responsible for filling out the MDS? How does the role of the LPN/LVN differ from the RN with regard to the resident assessments for the MDS?

CHAPTER 4

COMMON HEALTH PROBLEMS OF RESIDENTS IN NURSING HOMES

OUTLINE

Falls
Pressure Ulcers
Cognitive Dysfunction
Malnutrition
Constipation
Diarrhea

ORGANIZATION AND CONTENT

Chapter 4 identifies the major health problems that the nurse is likely to encounter with nursing home residents. The physical, emotional, and economic consequences of the problems are explored. Prevention strategies are fully discussed for each of the problems. Chapters 3 and 4 provide the core definition of the population and of the health problems that nurses work with in the nursing home setting.

For shorter courses, the focus should be on the assessment, prevention, and treatment of the common problems of elderly residents. Practical suggestions for the management of difficult resident behaviors may be supplemented by suggesting a review of the principles of therapeutic communication. Ethical implications for various prevention strategies, such as restraints, should be discussed.

For longer courses, the focus should include a complete review of nutritional assessment, the nursing care of residents with tube feedings, and the special care needed for residents with either partial or total parenteral nutrition. Ethical implications for the use of tube feeding and the withholding of food and fluids should be discussed.

INTERNET RESOURCES (BE SURE TO CHECK EACH ADDRESS.)

Tactilitics, Inc.

RNPlus
http://www.rnplus.com
A commercial site that contains an excellent review of falls, from risk assessment through interventions. Also contains a large bibliography and links to other sources.

National Pressure Ulcer Advisory Panel (NPUAP)
http://www.npuap.org/prevent
The NPUAP first convened in November 1987 with the mission of providing leadership in pressure ulcer prevention. Contains an excellent review of pressure ulcers, from risk assessment through interventions. Also contains a large bibliography and links to other sites.

IncontiNet
Incontinence on the Internet
http://incontinet.com/articles/AHCPR/overview.html
Describes itself as the Internet's largest resource on incontinence. Contains an excellent review of incontinence, from risk assessment through interventions. Also contains a large bibliography and links to other sites.

Alzheimer's Association
http://www.alz.org/lib/lists/Top.html
Contains excellent bibliographic resources for a variety of issues with Alzheimer's disease.

Rush University Alzheimer's Disease Center
http:/www.rush.edu/Med/RADC/index.html
Contains a variety of resources for professionals and families dealing with Alzheimer's disease.

University of Pittsburgh
http://www.pitt.edu/~rkrst3/homepage.html
Contains excellent assessment information on malnutrition in the elderly.

Pharminfonet
http://pharminfo.com/pubs/msb/constip.html
A commercial site that contains excellent information about pharmacology and various diseases. Has an excellent summary of constipation and its treatment.

CRITICAL THINKING EXERCISES

Group Assignments

Ask learners to:

- Select one common health problem for nursing home residents, and develop a preventive care plan based on several references from the Internet.
- Develop a list of community resources, including support groups, for families.who are dealing with an incontinent elder or an elder who is dealing with Alzheimer's disease.

Discussion Items

Ask learners to:

- Describe physiologic changes in the elderly that place them at risk for falls.
- Discuss environmental changes that the nurse can suggest to make living spaces safer for elders.
- Describe physiologic changes in the elderly that place them at risk for pressure ulcers.
- Compare malnutrition in younger and older nursing home residents.

Case Study

Present the following case study to the class. After giving students the information, break them into groups for discussion. Ask one person to be the recorder, one to be the timekeeper, one to present the group's decisions to the class, and one to ensure that all members contribute to the discussion.

> Mrs. Anita Hill is a 74-year-old white woman who has recently moved to her daughter's home. During a routine physical examination, her daughter mentions that her mother seems slower and more sedentary than she did a year ago. Mrs. Hill becomes dizzy on a walk to the mailbox. As a result, she falls on the uneven cement sidewalk. She is unable to get up and reports hearing a sound like a dry branch breaking when she fell. Mrs. Hill had surgery to repair her broken hip. A few days after the surgery, Mrs. Hill's nurse notes that she is disoriented to place and time. She is unable to state where she is or what time of day it is.

Group 1
- What questions might you ask Mrs. Hill about her activity?
- What laboratory tests would you like to see ordered for Mrs. Hill?

Group 2
- What advice could you have given Mrs. Hill's daughter that might have

- prevented Mrs. Hill's fall?
- What data in Mrs. Hill's history indicate that she was at risk for injury from a fall?

Group 3
- What other assessments should Mrs. Hill's nurse make?
- What interventions might help Mrs. Hill remain oriented to place and time?

SUGGESTED SUPPLEMENTAL MATERIALS

When discussing the ethical implications of restraints, tube feeding, and the withholding of food and fluid, have several copies of the American Nurses' Association *Code for Nurses* available for student reference. Additional materials might include a copy of the state and/or federal regulations regarding the use of restraints.

AMERICAN NURSES' ASSOCIATION
CODE FOR NURSES

1. The nurse provides services with respect for human dignity and the uniqueness of the client unrestricted by considerations of social or economic status, personal attributes, or the nature of the health problem.
2. The nurse safeguards the client's right to privacy by judiciously protecting information of a confidential nature.
3. The nurse acts to safeguard the client and the public when health care and safety are affect by the incompetent, unethical, or illegal practice of any person.
4. The nurse assumes responsibility and accountability for individual nursing judgments and actions.
5. The nurse maintains competence in nursing.
6. The nurse exercises informed judgment and uses individual competence and qualifications as criteria in seeking consultation, accepting responsibilities, and delegating nursing activities to others.
7. The nurse participates in activities that contribute to the ongoing development of the profession's body of knowledge.
8. The nurse participates in the profession's efforts to implement and improve standards of nursing.
9. The nurse participates in the profession's efforts to establish and maintain conditions of employment conducive to high-quality nursing care.
10. The nurse participates in the profession's efforts to protect the public from misinformation and misrepresentation and to maintain the integrity

of nursing.
11.. The nurse collaborates with members of the health professions and other citizens in promoting community and national efforts to meet the health needs of the public.

CHAPTER FIVE

MEDICATION USE IN THE ELDERLY

OUTLINE

Factors Contributing to Multiple Drug Use Among the Elderly
Pharmacokinetics and the Elderly
Common Complications of Drug Therapy in the Elderly
Pain Management in the Elderly
Infusion Therapy in Nursing Homes
Unnecessary Drugs
Self-Administration of Drugs
Medication Administration for Tips

ORGANIZATION AND CONTENT

Chapter 5 identifies the major concerns about medication administration specific to the elderly. Drawing on the physiologic changes itemized in Chapter 3, learners are guided through the impact these changes have on drug utilization. Information is also given regarding pain and infusion therapy that are specific to the elderly.

For shorter courses, learners can be directed to review a fundamentals of nursing text for pain assessment, medication administration techniques, and infusion therapy guidelines. The focus should highlight pain management strategies, both pharmacologic and nonpharmacologic.

For longer courses, the focus should include a detailed discussion of the differences in infusion therapy in the nursing home setting compared with an acute care setting. It would also be important to highlight the issue of unnecessary drugs and the nurse's responsibilty for monitoring residents' responses to their drug regimen.

INTERNET RESOURCES (BE SURE TO CHECK EACH ADDRESS.)

U.S. Pharmacopeia
http://www.usp.org/did/elements.htm
This Internet site contains a drug information area that permits health care

workers to determine the essential patient teaching information for drugs. There is also a limited permission to copy information form for clients.

CRITICAL THINKING EXERCISES

Group Assignment

Give each group of learners a commonly administered drug, such as digoxin, and ask learners to:

- Identify how aging affects that drug's absorption and excretion.
- Identify what information the resident and family should have about the drug.
- Predict which of the listed adverse reactions are more likely to occur with the elderly.

Have the groups share the information with one another by sending one student from each group to a different group to gather their information. That student then comes back to the home group and shares the information with the home group. Each student thus has the chance to be the "expert" in the new group and add needed information to the home group.

Discussion Items

Ask leaners to:

- State the rationale for obtaining a detailed drug history on an elder.
- Identify three physiologic changes with aging that may affect drug utilization.
- Describe the assessments that are appropriate when an 87-year-old nursing home resident tells the nurse that she has increasing pain in her hips.
- Identify some nonpharmacologic interventions that the nurse may employ to help residents manage pain.
- Identify interventions that minimize complications in the elderly receiving intravenous therapy.

Case Study

Present the following case study to the class. After giving students the information, break them into groups for discussion. Ask one person to be the recorder, one to be the timekeeper, one to present the group's decisions to the class, and one student to assure that all members contribute to the discussion.

> Mrs. Chang Yi, aged 78, was admitted to the nursing home 2 weeks ago following a hospital admission for congestive heart failure and chronic renal failure. She is 4 feet 10 inches tall and currently weighs 89 pounds. Her vital signs have been stable, and she has lost approximately 2 pounds since admission. In addition to several drugs to manage her chronic renal failure, Mrs. Yi is taking digoxin 0.125 mg PO every other day and furosemide (Lasix) 20 mg PO BID to manage her congestive heart failure. The geriatric nursing assistant (GNA) working with Mrs. Yi tells you that Mrs. Yi has refused to eat both breakfast and lunch and that she seems listless. A review of Mrs. Yi's daily intake sheets show that she has routinely taken in 700 to 750 mL of the 1000 mL of fluid per day that she is allowed. She has also eaten less than 50 percent of her meals each day since admission.

- *Group 1*
  What data indicate that Mrs. Yi is at risk for complications of her drug therapy?
- *Group 2*
  What assessments should the nurse make?
- *Group 3*
  What interventions, if any, might the nurse might implement at this time?
- *Group 4*
  What laboratory tests can the nurse anticipate that the physician may order?

CHAPTER 6

ACUTE ILLNESSES AND HEALTH EMERGENCIES

OUTLINE

Acute Infections
Fluid Imbalances
Common Electrolyte Imbalances
Diabetic Emergencies
Myocardial Infarction
Vascular Emergencies

ORGANIZATION AND CONTENT

Chapter 6 describes the commonly occurring acute illnesses and health emergencies in long term care residents. Both prevention and intervention strategies are emphasized.

For shorter courses, learners focus on both the common assessments for each health problem and the appropriate intervention strategies.

For longer courses, learners should further explore the prevention strategies and monitoring activities that must be undertaken to safeguard residents.

INTERNET RESOURCES (BE SURE TO CHECK EACH ADDRESS.)

Avicenna
http://www.avicenna.com
An excellent source for disease-specific information through the National Library of Medicine's Medline.

CRITICAL THINKING EXERCISES

Group Assignment

Ask groups of learners to go on-line and find information on a health problem.

Each group should select a different health problem. Learners should be directed to find two or three articles that focus on either assessment or interventions to treat the health problem. Learners could also be asked to evaluate the articles' usefulness and whether they would recommend that others read the articles.

Discussion Items

Ask learners to:

- List two general measures to prevent acute infections in long term care residents.
- Describe at least three assessments and three nursing interventions for respiratory and urinary tract infections.
- Describe at least eight common assessment findings that indicate fluid imbalance in elderly residents.
- Identify the most common electrolyte imbalances in elderly residents and two assessment findings that would indicate the imbalances.
- Identify two common diabetic emergencies and describe the assessment and interventions for each emergency.
- Describe the assessment findings that would indicate a myocardial infarction rather than angina in elderly residents.
- Identify four assessment findings that would help differentiate between arterial and venous occlusions.

Case Studies

Present the following case studies to the class. After giving learners the information, break them into groups for discussion. Ask one person to be the recorder, one to be the timekeeper, one to present the group's decisions to the class, and one to ensure that all members contribute to the discussion.

Case No. 1

Mrs. Janice Wilson, aged 76, has congestive heart failure following a myocardial infarction 3 years ago. Generally she is able to meet her hygiene needs and walks about 50 feet to the dining room for meals. The geriatric nursing assistant (GNA) reports that Mrs. Wilson refuses go to the dining room for lunch today, saying that she's "too tuckered out." The GNA also reports that Mrs. Wilson has refused to go to the dining room for the last three days. During an assessment, the nurse notes that Mrs. Wilson's ankles are now puffy with 3+ pitting edema, she is dyspneic on exertion, and has gained 3 pounds since she was weighed 6 days ago.

Group 1
- Describe other assessment data that the nurse should gather from Mrs. Wilson and her medical record.

Group 2
- Describe the medications that are most likely ordered for Mrs. Wilson. What additional medications would the nurse expect to be ordered? What teaching should the nurse plan for Mrs. Wilson?

Group 3
- Identify two priority nursing diagnoses for Mrs. Wilson. Present at least two nursing interventions for each diagnosis.

Group 4
- What evidence would the nurse use to determine the success of the nursing interventions for Mrs. Wilson?

Case No. 2

Mrs. Kay Wendis, aged 78, has type II diabetes mellitus, hypertension, and left-sided paralysis from a stroke. The geriatric nursing assistant (GNA) reports that Mrs. Wendis has had four large watery stools today and that her tongue and mouth are dry and cracked. The GNA also reports that Mrs. Wendis has complained of abdominal pain today. A finger-stick glucose test reveals that Mrs. Wendis's blood sugar is 780 mg/dL.

Group 1
- Identify the most likely cause for Mrs. Wendis' symptoms. What other physical assessment findings would help to confirm the cause of symptoms?

Group 2
- Describe the likely medical treatment to be ordered for Mrs. Wendis. Is it likely that Mrs. Wendis will require further treatment in a hospital?

Group 3
- Identify two priority nursing diagnoses for Mrs. Wendis. Present at least two interventions for each diagnosis.

Group 4
- What evidence would the nurse use to determine the success of the nursing interventions for Mrs. Wendis?

CHAPTER 7

DOCUMENTATION REQUIREMENTS IN THE NURSING HOME

OUTLINE

Comprehensive Resident Care Plan
Clinical Pathway
Progress Notes
Activity and Treatment Records
Incident Report

ORGANIZATION AND CONTENT

Chapter 7 describes documentation required for comprehensive care planning in long term care facilities. Descriptions of the purposes for progress notes, styles of charting, and various special assessment sheets are given. Having sample documentation forms, such as a resident progress note, special skin assessment record, medication administration record, and incident report, are very helpful. Forms can be distributed or shown on an overhead transparency while discussing their use.

For shorter courses, learners should focus on the legal requirements for adequate documentation, the styles of charting, and the various special purpose records in the long term care setting.

For longer courses, learners should be further directed to the benefits and disadvantages of clinical pathways versus traditional comprehensive resident care plans and the use of progress notes for documentation of quality care.

CRITICAL THINKING EXERCISES

Group Assignment

Provide groups of learners with the following sample resident information. Ask each group to format their progress note as one of the following: a narrative note, a PIE note, or a focus note (DARE). Each group should present their sample note. Learners should be asked to identify the advantages and disadvantages of each note.

SAMPLE RESIDENT INFORMATION

1. An elderly resident was found on the floor next to her bed at 0645 by the geriatric nursing assistant (GNA).
2. Vital signs at 0647 were T 98.8 degrees Fahrenheit, P 88, R 22, BP 146/98.
3. The resident had no complaints of pain when questioned.
4. The resident is able to move freely.
5. There is a reddened area on left lateral thigh about 5 inches from the knee, but no other apparent bruises or breaks in the skin.
6. The resident says that she was on her way to the bathroom when she got dizzy and sat on the floor.
7. No one saw the resident between rounds at 0630, when she appeared to be sleeping, and the time she was found on the floor.
8. The supervisor was notified at 0650.
9. A message was left for the resident's physician at 0652.

Discussion Items

Ask learners to:

- Discuss how a comprehensive resident care plan differs from a nursing care plan in an acute care setting.
- Describe how a clinical pathway differs from a nursing care plan.
- Describe the economic importance of progress notes, both from the residents' and the facility's view.
- Describe how focus notes differ from PIE notes.
- Identify the important legal guidelines for completing an incident report.

Case Study

Present the following case study to the class. After giving learners the information, break them into groups for discussion. Ask one person to be the recorder, one to be the timekeeper, one to present the group's decisions to the class, and one to ensure that all members contribute to the discussion.

> Mr. Harold Smith's son, Joe, approached the nurses' station to speak with his father's nurse. Joe Smith expressed concern that there were several bruises and breaks in the skin surface on his father's arms that had not been present when he visited his father yesterday. Joe Smith was respectful but determined to "get to the bottom of this situation."

- ***Group 1***
  What information should the nurse expect to find on Mr. Harold Smith's progress note? Is there information that should NOT be on Mr. Smith's progress note?
  Group 2
- What information should the nurse expect to see on any incident report form? What, if anything, should be OMITTED from the form?
  Group 3
- Who must be informed of a resident's untoward event, such as a fall? Does the fact that Mr. Smith is competent make any difference in how the nurse responds to Mr. Joe Smith?
  Group 4
- How should the conversation with Mr. Joe Smith be documented?

CHAPTER 8

HEALTH PROTECTION AND PROMOTION IN THE NURSING HOME

OUTLINE

Healthy People 2000
Resident Education

ORGANIZATION AND CONTENT

Chapter 8 describes the teaching-learning process with the variations appropriate to the long term care resident.

For shorter courses, learners should focus on the teaching-learning process as it is affected by aging and on the interventions that are appropriate for the elderly resident. Health promotion should be addressed in general.

For longer courses, learners should also explore the interventions that are appropriate for health promotion for specific health problems.

INTERNET RESOURCES (BE SURE TO CHECK EACH ADDRESS.)

Healthy People 2000
http:www.crisny/health/us/health7.html
Full text description of the *Healthy People 2000* agenda, with resources listed for further information on various priority issues.

Dietary Guidelines for Americans
Http://www.nal.usda.gov/fnic/Dietary/9dietgui.htm
Full-text description of the elements of a healthy diet with tables and statistics. Full color. Easy reading. An excellent teaching resource.

American Cancer Society
http://www.cancer.org/frames/html
Home page for the American Cancer Society. An excellent resource for locating teaching materials.

CA: A Cancer Journal for Clinicians
http://www.lrpub.com/ca
Full-text articles with information from current research. Articles cover a wide variety of cancer topics. Excellent reference source.

CRITICAL THINKING EXERCISES

Group Assignment

Ask groups of learners to develop a teaching plan for one of the following residents:

1. An-86-year old man with left-sided paralysis who has poor oral hygiene.
2. A 72-year-old woman with osteoporosis and poor nutrition who has fallen several times.
3. A 45-year-old man who is post–head trauma and frequently makes frankly sexual remarks to the geriatric nursing assistants (GNAs).
4. A 68-year-old woman with recent bilateral above-the-knee amputations who wants to cook her own meals.

Learners should be asked to identify the additional assessment data that they feel would help them develop the teaching plan. Learners should also be asked to identify the outcome behaviors by which goal achievement can be measured for each resident. Each group should share their desired additional assessment data, outcome behaviors, and brief teaching plan with the whole group.

Discussion Items

Ask learners to:

- Draw a picture to represent the relationship between health promotion and health protection.
- Describe how the teaching-learning process and nursing process are alike and different.
- Identify at least three effects that aging has on the teaching-learning process.
- Describe at least four teaching interventions that might help the elderly resident to learn.

Case Study

Present the following case study to the class. After giving learners the information, break them into groups for discussion. Ask one person to be the recorder, one to be the timekeeper, one to present the group's decisions to the class, and one to ensure that all members contribute to the discussion.

> Mrs. Muriel Garcia, aged 72, has been admitted to the extended stay facility following surgery for a permanent colostomy 3 days ago. Mrs. Garcia needs to learn to manage her colostomy before she can be discharged home. At the present time, she is refusing to look at the stoma during dressing changes. When asked to participate in the colostomy care, she cries and states, "I can't, I can't. Leave me alone! Just do what you have to do, and leave me alone!" She refuses to go to the dining room and lies in bed with the sheet pulled over her head.

Group 1
- Identify factors that may be interfering with Mrs. Garcia's ability to participate in her colostomy care. What interventions should be tried to improve Mrs. Garcia's ability to learn to manage her colostomy?

Group 2
- List the skills Mrs. Garcia must master in order to successfully manage her colostomy? How can those skills be measured?

Group 3
- Identify the knowledge that Mrs. Garcia must have to prevent complications from occurring with her colostomy. How can the nurse be certain that Mrs. Garcia knows the prevention information?

Group 4
- Assume that Mrs. Garcia had surgery because of cancer of the colon. What health practices should the nurse teach her for health promotion.

CHAPTER 9

SUBACUTE CARE

OUTLINE

Definitions of Subacute Care
Standards and Regulations Governing Subacute Care
Settings for Subacute Care
Types of Subacute Patients
The Role of the Nurse in Subacute Care
Internal Case Management in Subacute Care
Future of Subacute Care

ORGANIZATION AND CONTENT

Chapter 9 defines and describes subacute or transitional care. The regulatory standards, settings, and types of subacute patients are surveyed. The role of the nurse in subacute care is discussed, and the role of the nurse as case manager is explored.

For shorter courses, the learner should become familiar with the concept of subacute care, the types of patients in subacute care, and the role and qualifications required of the nurse in a transitional setting.

For longer courses, the learner should be directed to the role of the nurse as case manager. The use of clinical pathways in subacute settings should also be highlighted.

INTERNET RESOURCES (BE SURE TO CHECK EACH ADDRESS.)

Medical Rehabilitation Services and Health Care Policy
http://www.intr.net/nrhrc/t2subact.html
This resource provides an extensive bibliography on subacute care. The database also permits searches for specific issues such as case management in subacute care.

CRITICAL THINKING EXERCISES

Group Assignment

Ask groups of learners to go on-line and find an article in the Medical Rehabilitation Services and Health Care Policy bibliography. If time is limited, the instructor might do the search, select several articles, and ask groups of students to report their information after reading the articles.

Discussion Items

Ask learners to:

- Describe how subacute care and acute care are alike and how they differ.
- Identify how subacute care units are evaluated to ensure that quality care is being delivered.
- Compare and contrast three different types of subacute care settings.
- Describe the nursing skills that are required of nursing staff working in a subacute unit.
- Explain how the role of nurse as coordinator of care is affected by case management.

Case Study

Present the following case study to the class. After giving learners the information, break them into groups for discussion. Ask one person to be the recorder, one to be the timekeeper, one to present the group's decisions to the class, and one to ensure that all members contribute to the discussion.

> Mrs. Henrietta O'Halloran, aged 76, is being admitted to the hospital today for a total knee replacement. She is a widow and lives alone in her two-story home. Her daughter, Kate, lives 10 miles away with her husband and four children. Kate's home is too small to have her mother stay with her after surgery, and Kate's young, school-age children make it impossible for her to go and stay with her mother in her mother's home. Both realize that Mrs. O'Halloran will need active physical therapy and a period of time before she is able to meet her activities of daily living comfortably or to manage her home.
>
> ***Group 1***
> - Determine what type of subacute care might best meet Mrs. O'Halloran's needs. List the considerations that made you choose that type of subacute care.
>
> ***Group 2***

- Identify some concerns that Mrs. O'Halloran might have about subacute care.
  Group 3
- Identify some concerns Mrs. O'Halloran's daughter might have about subacute care.
  Group 4
- Does the role of the nurse on the orthopedic unit in the acute care setting differ from the role of the nurse in the subacute care setting? Will different skills be required for managing Mrs. O'Halloran in each setting?

CHAPTER 10

PHILOSOPHY AND STRUCTURE OF THE NURSING HOME

OUTLINE

Role of Ownership
Role of the Nursing Home Administrator
Role of Clinical Departments
Role of Nonclinical Departments

ORGANIZATION AND CONTENT

Chapter 10 describes the organizational structure of long term care facilities. Learners should be reminded that the same functions that are necessary for safe care in acute care settings are essential in long term care settings. There is a tension between attempting to maintain a homelike environment while ensuring a safe care environment for all residents.

For shorter courses, learners should be directed to the similarities and differences in the roles of the clinical and nonclinical departments compared with those in acute care settings.

For longer courses, learners should further explore the impact of the type of ownership on the long term care facility. In addition, the role and responsibilities of the nursing home administrator should be discussed.

INTERNET RESOURCES

Nursing Home Administrators' Curriculum
http://www.mankato.msus.edu/dept/gero/NursHomeLic.html
This resource clearly lists the course work needed to qualify for a nursing home administrator's license in Minnesota. Similar requirements exist in each state.

A Day in the Life of a Nursing Home Medical Director
http://www.ascu.buffalo.edu/~drstall/nhmdrole.txt
An outline of a lecture on the role of the nursing home medical director. Interesting reading, and the outline gives a good indication of the complexity and the diversity of the role of the nursing home medical director.

CRITICAL THINKING EXERCISES

Group Assignment

Ask groups of learners to:

Discussion Items

Ask learners to:
- List advantages and disadvantages of for-profit, not-for-profit, and government-owned long term care facilities.
- Identify the qualifications generally required of nursing home administrators.
- Describe how physician services differ in long term care settings from those in acute care settings.
- Describe the duties of the staff development coordinator.

Case Study

Present the following case study to the class. After giving learners the information, break them into groups for discussion. Ask one person to be the recorder, one to be the timekeeper, one to present the group's decisions to the class, and one to ensure that all members contribute to the discussion.

Assume that you are a newly employed nurse at XWY Manor, a nursing home. You started orientation 3 days ago.

Group 1
- A resident's family member approaches the nurses' station and asks you to explain to them "just exactly what does the nursing home administrator do?" What would you tell them?

Group 2
- While answering a resident's call light, you discover that the toilet in the room is running continuously. After toggling the flush handle, the toilet continues to run. Which department would you call? If the toilet over ran onto the floor? Are there other measures you should take?

Group 3
- During a chart review, you note that a resident's weight has dropped 6 pounds in 2 weeks. What interventions are appropriate? Which departments, if any, should be notified?

Group 4

- A resident's family member invites you to defend the quality of care given at XWZ Manor. To which department or function might you turn for information? Are there other issues that might be explored with the family member?

CHAPTER 11

ORGANIZATION AND FUNCTION OF THE NURSING DEPARTMENT

OUTLINE

Director of Nursing
Assistant Director of Nursing
Quality Improvement Coordinator
Nursing Supervisor
Minimum Data Set Supervisor
Unit Coordinator
Charge Nurse
Staff Nurse
Geriatric Nursing Assistant/Aide
Certified Medicine Aide
Care/Case Manager

ORGANIZATION AND CONTENT

Chapter 11 briefly describes the roles and functions of the nursing department in a nursing home. Specific areas covered are the role of the nursing director and assistant director, and the duties of the various care or function coordinators.

For shorter courses, the learner should be directed to the specific roles of the nursing director, the unit coordinator, nursing supervisor, and the various nursing service personnel on the nursing units. The roles of the various care or function coordinators should also be briefly examined.

For longer courses, the learner should be directed to the roles of the quality improvement coordinator, the nursing supervisor, the Minimum Data Set (MDS) coordinator, and the care/case manager. The role of the unit nurse on each of these functions should be explored in detail.

INTERNET RESOURCES (Be sure to check each address.)

Hospitals and Nursing Homes Need Changes in the Mix of Nursing Personnel
A report by the National Research Council

http://www.edu/onpi/pr/jan96/nurse.html
The reference is a report by the Institute of Medicine that describes the needed mix of personnel in hospitals and nursing homes.

CRITICAL THINKING EXERCISES

Group Assignment

Ask groups of learners to read the National Research Council report listed previously. Each group should focus on one area: acute care, nursing home care, or reduction of injury and stress.

Discussion Items

Ask learners to:

- List the suggestions made by the article.
- Develop a plan to validate the cost of implementing the suggested changes.
- If possible, develop a plan to evaluate the savings estimated by the writers of the article.

Case Study

Present the following case study to the class. After giving learners the information, break them into groups for discussion. Ask one person to be the recorder, one to be the timekeeper, one to present the group's decisions to the class, and one to ensure that all members contribute to the discussion.

> Lowell Manor Nursing Home has 135 residents divided evenly on three wings. In addition to the nursing home administrator, the facility has a director of nursing, assistant director of nursing, three RN nurse supervisors, three RN unit coordinators, 20 LPNs, 29 geriatric nursing assistants, 3 geriatric medicine aides, plus an RN quality assurance coordinator, and a part-time RN MDS coordinator.
>
> *Group 1*
> - Assuming that the resident care requirements are roughly equal on all three wings, develop a staffing plan with the listed personnel. The director, assistant director, function coordinators (quality improvement [QI] and MDS), and the nursing supervisors are not available for resident care. Be sure to include all shifts for days.

Group 2
- Diagram an organizational chart for the nursing service of Lowell Manor Nursing Home.
- How does your chart reflect your expected channels of communication?

Group 3
- With only three RN supervisors, there will be times when a supervisor is not immediately available. What provisions must be made for that occurrence?
- What does your state board of nursing regulations say about supervision by RNs and by LPNs?

Group 4
- How do the roles of the QI coordinator and the MDS coordinator assist the nursing staff to give care?
- To whom do the QI and MDS coordinators report?

CHAPTER 12

ROLE OF THE CHARGE NURSE

OUTLINE

Staffing Patterns
Roles and Responsibilities of the Charge Nurse

ORGANIZATION AND CONTENT

Chapter 12 briefly describes the role of charge nurse in long term care. A discussion of staffing patterns and specific role responsibilities offer detailed information on role requirements and skills.

For shorter courses, learners should be directed to the actual role requirements, such as shift reporting, staff assignment, the legal issues involved with supervision and delegation, and conflict management.

For longer courses, the learner should be directed additionally to team building, communication, and leadership styles. The learner should also know what role they are to play in the evaluation of the performance of other team members.

INTERNET RESOURCES (BE SURE TO CHECK EACH ADDRESS.)

Staff Assignment
Assignment of Nursing Care for Patients
http://www.cc.nih.gov/nursing/assignnc.html
The resource identifies the elements that must be considered when charge nurses make out patient care assignments. A very complete, compact outline of issues.

Continuing Education (CE)
On-line CE Credit
http://www.ajn.org/CE/CEsOnline.cfm
http://www.aorn.org/JOURNAL/homestudy.htm
http://www.ce-web.com/
http://www.learnwell.org/~edu/rnonline.shtml
http://www.nccn.net/~wwithin/homstud.htm

http://www.nurseweek.com/ce/cew3.html
http://www.springnet.com/ce/ceartlst.htm

Other Internet CE Resources
Videotape: http://www.geriatricvideo.com/
Audiotape: http://www.son.washington.edu/~cne/images/is.html
E-mail: http://www.nursing.ab.umd.edu/offices/opds/ce/bdceu.html
(These resources were listed in the June issue of *Nursing97*, p 20.)

CRITICAL THINKING EXERCISES

Group Assignment

Ask groups of learners to go on-line with one of the CE references listed. Each group should select a different reference source. Each group should describe the CE programs and credits that the reference source has available. Help the groups by structuring a worksheet for them to complete. Suggestions for the worksheet include:

- What is the reference source used (full Internet address)?
- What CE programs are available?
- Can credit be transmitted on-line?
- What is the CE provider's name?
- Other comments that students think their classmates should know, for example, ease of moving through the CE offering, graphics, and so forth.

Each group of students should complete the worksheet and be ready to share their information with the whole group.

Discussion Items

Ask learners to:

- Compare and contrast the position of charge nurse with the position of head nurse.
- List items that should be included in a complete shift report.
- State clearly how delegation and supervision differ.
- Describe the elements needed to safely delegate a nursing function to another staff member.
- Give examples of each of the five resolutions to conflict.

Case Study

Present the following case study to the class. After giving learners the information, break them into groups for discussion. Ask one person to be the recorder, one to be the timekeeper, one to present the group's decisions to the class, and one to ensure that all members contribute to the discussion.

> Hannah Gruen, RN, is the day charge nurse for her unit in the long term care facility. She has two LPNs and four geriatric nursing assistants, as well as the unit secretary, as staff today. Ms. Gruen listened to the shift report from the off-going night nurse and has learned that two of the residents will need extra supervision today because one resident suffered a seizure at 0300 and the second resident fell after toileting and possibly struck her head. The resident is confused and restless this morning.
>
> Both residents are on the same wing, so Ms. Gruen assigned one LPN team leader three GNAs for the day to account for the increased observation and care, and the other LPN one GNA. Ms. Gruen specified that each of the two residents should be checked carefully every hour and any untoward finding reported. At 1315 while making rounds, Ms. Gruen found the post-fall resident sitting on the floor with a severe droop to the left side of her face. Ms. Gruen checked the frequent note sheet and saw that neither the LPN nor any GNA had checked the resident since 1100.
>
> Ms. Gruen finds the LPN, who states she asked one of the GNAs to check the resident at 1200 because she was feeding another resident. The GNA acknowledges that the LPN asked her to check the resident, but she was "too busy helping out on the other wing because they're so short today" to check the resident as requested, but that she had asked another GNA to check the resident "when she had time."

Group One
- What elements must be considered when making an assignment?
- Did Ms. Gruen make an appropriate staff assignment?

Group Two
- What elements must be considered when delegating nursing care?
- Did Ms. Gruen make an appropriate delegation to the LPN?

Group Three
- Did the LPN make an appropriate delegation to the GNA?
- What supervisory responsibilities did the LPN and Ms. Gruen have?

Group Four
- How could communication between Ms. Gruen and her staff been improved so that the resident was observed as desired.
- What effect did usual staffing patterns have on the GNAs?

CHAPTER 13

THE SURVEY PROCESS

OUTLINE

The Survey Team
Survey Preparation
Entrance Conference and Orientation Tour
Resident Sampling
Quality Assessments
Information Analysis and Decision making
Exit Conference
Follow-up Surveys
Voluntary Accreditation
Role of the Nurse

ORGANIZATION AND CONTENT

Chapter 13 briefly describes the long term care facility inspection process from preinspection through follow-up procedures. The state and federal regulations and the uses of the survey report are also described.

For shorter courses, the learner should be directed to the steps in the process and the types of information the surveyors are seeking during that part of the process. The learner should also be familiar with the role of the nurse in the survey process.

For longer courses, the learner should be further directed to the follow-up elements of information analysis as well as processes. The role of voluntary accreditation in financial reimbursement should be explored.

INTERNET RESOURCES (BE SURE TO CHECK EACH ADDRESS.)

Joint Commission on Accreditation of Hospitals (JCAHO) Survey Information
http://www.jchao.org/acr_info/ltc.html#1_6
This resource describes the elements of the JCAHO survey requirements for long term care.

Enforcement Rules for Nursing Facilities
http://www.rbvdnr.com/health/alert.htm
The resource explains the Health Care Finance Administration penalties for poor survey reports.

CRITICAL THINKING EXERCISES

Group Assignment

Ask groups of learners to role-play a nurse survey team member and a nursing home administrator during an unexpected survey visit. Each group should develop a list of observations that the survey team member might make with regard to determining patients' quality of life and the potential concerns of the facility administrator with regard to residents' rights.

Discussion Items

Ask learners to:
- List at least four general areas that survey team members will ask to observe.
- Compare and contrast the quality of care assessment and the quality of life assessment.
- Identify the specific items that would indicate to a surveyor that drug therapy has been appropriately ordered and monitored for a patient?
- Identify the specific items that would indicate to a surveyor that nutrition therapy has been appropriately ordered and monitored for a patient.
- Identify the items of information that are usually included in an exit interview.
- Identify at least two significant areas in which the JCAHO accreditation process and the state accreditation differ.
- Identify what information and skills a nurse must have that specifically relate to the survey process.

Case Study

Present the following case study to the class. After giving learners the information, break them into groups for discussion. Ask one person to be the recorder, one to be the timekeeper, one to present the group's decisions to the class, and one to ensure that all members contribute to the discussion.

> Guadalupe Lopez, LPN, has been working for the nursing home for a year. She has been assigned to give medications today on her unit.

During the early morning medication pass, Ms. Lopez is informed that the state survey team has suddenly arrived on site and that she should expect a surveyor to accompany her during her 1000 medication pass. Ms. Lopez has never participated in a survey and expresses great apprehension to her charge nurse.

Group 1
- How should the charge nurse respond to Ms. Lopez' concerns?
- Identify at least two concerns that Ms. Lopez might express.

Group 2
- Identify at least two areas that the surveyor will be observing while Ms. Lopez does her medication pass.
- What would indicate to the surveyor that an error in procedure has occurred? (Use material in the appendix on the operational standards for the medication pass).

Group 3
- What information should Ms. Lopez be familiar with in the event that the surveyor asks about a resident's drug therapy?
- Identify particular classes of drugs or particular drugs that require documentation beyond signing off the medication administration record.

Group 4
- How and when will the information gathered by the surveyor be presented to the facility?
- Identify what information is likely to be given when the information is reported to the facility.
- Because survey reports are widely distributed, how is the issue of confidentiality addressed by the survey team?

CHAPTER 14

THE QUALITY IMPROVEMENT PROCESS

OUTLINE

Quality Assurance and Assessment
Total Quality Management
Statistical Analysis
Staff Feedback

ORGANIZATION AND CONTENT

Chapter 14 briefly describes the key elements of the quality improvement process. Each element, such as the audit process, is examined through the information that the element adds to the understanding of the concept quality care. The chapter further describes the concept of total quality management and information analysis.

    For shorter courses, the learner should be directed to the quality assurance process, specifically the various elements of that process. Emphasis should be placed on the contribution that nurses make to setting quality-care standards and the monitoring process.

    For longer courses, the learner should be also directed to the concept of total quality management and the analytic requirements of the subelements of continuous quality improvement, which include risk management, performance management, and utilization review. The role of the nurse in these important functions should be emphasized.

INTERNET RESOURCES (BE SURE TO CHECK EACH ADDRESS.)

Continuous Quality Improvement
http://www.ftp.uth.tmc.edu/ut_general/admin_fn/cqi/research/tools/
A tool that outlines all areas of continuous quality improvement. One area is highlighted, and a detailed checklist is provided.

Risk Management
Back Strain in Nursing Homes: Index
http://www.wt.com.au/~dohswa/d_pubs/nursing/nurs_ind.htm

The reference provides an extensive resource list of articles and other learning materials to help educators put together learning programs to decrease back injury in nursing homes.

Performance Management
http://www.pw2.netcom.com/~pab_hart/cert4.htm
The reference provides information about the documentation necessary for the performance appraisal.

Utilization Review
Practice Pointer: What to Look for in Your State Utilization Review Law
http://www.apa.org/practice/pointer2.html
The reference details the concerns that professionals might have about state utilization review laws. Includes information on how disputes are settled.

CRITICAL THINKING EXERCISES

Group Assignment

Ask groups of learners to take a problem, such as pressure ulcers, use of restraints, overmedication, or undernutrition, and to develop a set of outcome standards to determine and/or correct the problem. Learners should be directed to focus on these questions:

- How do nurses determine that the problem exists?
- How do nurses determine that the problem has been resolved?

Each group should designate a recorder, timekeeper, and reporter.

Discussion Items

Ask learners to:

- Compare and contrast quality assessment with quality assurance.
- Give an example of a structure, a process, and an outcome standard.
- Compare and contrast prospective, concurrent, and retrospective audits.
- Give an example of an instrument used in a prospective, concurrent, and retrospective audit.
- Report on their attendance at an audit meeting. Reports should include what types of audit the committee (or person) was doing, what type of information was the audit gathering, and what action was proposed based on the information that was being gathered.

Case Study

Present the following case study to the class. After giving learners the information, break them into groups for discussion. Ask one person to be the recorder, one to be the timekeeper, one to present the group's decisions to the class, and one to ensure that all members contribute to the discussion.

> Harold Bateman, RN, has noticed that his elderly patients in the long term care facility seem to have had a higher than average number of fall injuries. Mr. Bateman mentioned his concern to the Quality Assurance Committee member on his unit.

Group 1
- Describe the type of information the committee will need to begin working on Mr. Bateman's concern?
- List all the resources that will need to be or could be assembled for the committee's use.

Group 2
- Assuming that Mr. Bateman is correct, that more fall injuries have occurred, discuss how the committee will attempt to determine the cause of the increased fall injuries.
- List all the possible causes for fall injuries and the documentation that will help to determine which of these causes might be the problem.

Group 3
- Assume that the committee has determined that a high staff turnover has resulted in a large number of new geriatric nursing assistants (GNAs) who lack experience with fall prevention.
- Develop a staff development program to help educate the GNAs in fall prevention. List specific points to be included in the education program.

Group 4
- Assume that a cause for the increased falls has been identified and that staff have had several planned educational experiences in fall prevention.
- Identify several outcome measures that will demonstrate that the cause and the educational plan were successful in preventing fall injuries.
- Discuss the plans that should be made to prevent a further occurrence of increased fall injuries.

CHAPTER 15

LEGAL AND ETHICAL ISSUES IN THE LONG TERM CARE SETTING

OUTLINE

Legal Aspects Related to Resident Care
Ethical Decision Making

ORGANIZATION AND CONTENT

Chapter 15 briefly describes the legal basis for nursing practice in long term care, including a discussion of malpractice. In addition, the nurse's ethical decision making is explored as it applies to common ethical dilemmas encountered in long term care.

For shorter courses, learners should be directed to the legal basis for nursing practice, the process of ethical decision making, the ANA *Code for Nurses,* and the common ethical issues dealt with in long term care.

For longer courses, the learner should also explore the implications of labor relations and the legal basis for nursing practice among various levels of nursing personnel.

INTERNET RESOURCES (BE SURE TO CHECK EACH ADDRESS.)

Ethical Resources
http://www.ccme-mac4.bsd.uchicago.edy/ccme.html

Consumer Information Sources
http://www.hospice-cares.com/cons.html
http://www.lastacts.org

Other Learning Resources
End-of Life Care: Ethical Dimensions
Glaxo-Wellcome Continuing Nursing Education videotape (GNE015) and monograph (GNE017)

Available from a Glaxo-Wellcome representative. Call 800-824-2896 for ordering information.
The videotape and monograph are excellent resources for a discussion of end-of-life issues. The monograph also lists several excellent further resources for ethical decision making.

CRITICAL THINKING EXERCISES

Group Assignment (Also Known as a "Structured Controversy")

Ask pairs of learners to read: Francis, B. (1990). Walking a tightrope. *Nursing90*(February), 69. Before giving the learners the information to read, delete the last section of the article titled "The Consequences." Any other brief article that clearly presents an ethical dilemma and a decision-making process may be selected.

- Assign one learner in each pair to collect and present information to support the position that the nurse acted ethically. Ask the second learner to collect and present information that the nurse did not act ethically.
- Have each learner spend some time preparing his or her case, and then have each pair present his or her argument and facts to the opposing member of the pair.
- Require each learner to listen carefully and to note any faults with the argument from the opposition.
- Have each member attempts to rebute the position taken by the opposing member.
- Finally, have each member arrive at a consensus position with supporting arguments.

Case Study

Present the following case study to the class. After giving learners the information, break them into groups for discussion. Ask one person to be the recorder, one to be the timekeeper, one to present the group's decisions to the class, and one to ensure that all members contribute to the discussion.

> Mrs. Alvira Thomas, aged 75, is sitting by her husband's bedside crying when the nurse makes early morning rounds. Mr. Thomas, aged 73, suffered a massive cerebrovascular accident 4 days ago and has been in a deep coma since that time. When questioned by the nurse, Mrs. Thomas states that the physician said to her that Mr. Thomas is highly unlikely to get any better and that she needs to make a decision about what she

wants done if Mr. Thomas gets worse. She further tells the nurse that she is terribly confused and has no idea what to do. She asks the nurse what to do.

Group 1
- Identify what information Mrs. Thomas and her family might require in order to make a decision about resuscitation.

Group 2
- Identify the role that the nurse has as patient advocate for Mr. Thomas and for Mrs. Thomas and her family. Use the ANA *Code for Nurses* to identify the role of the nurse.

Group 3
- Identify other health care professionals or helping professionals that serve as resources for Mrs. Thomas and her family as they make their decision.

Group 4
- Identify the emotions that Mrs. Thomas and her family are likely to demonstrate. Plan one or two strategies to help Mrs. Thomas and her family to cope with those emotions.

TEST BANK

Chapter 1

1.
Mr. Hal Jensen, aged 96, lives at home with his wife. Although Mr. Jensen has several chronic health problems, both he and his wife enjoy their gardening and visits from their many children and their families. Mr. Jensen is:
A. Unusual for a middle old man
B. Usual for a middle old man
C. Unusual for an old old man
D. Usual for an old old man

2.
The percentage of adults over the age of 65 who may spend some part of their lives in a nursing home is:
A. 5 percent to 15 percent
B. 30 percent to 40 percent
C. 50 percent to 55 percent
D. 80 percent to 85 percent

3.
During a routine blood pressure check, Mrs. Mary Higgins, aged 72, tells the nurse that she is afraid of becoming dependent and having to live in a nursing home. Before responding, Mrs. Higgins's nurse needs to know that:
A. From 30 percent to 40 percent of people over age 65 are in relatively good health
B. About 23 percent of the U.S. population is over age 65
C. Only about 5 percent of people over age 65 are living in nursing homes
D. From 50 percent to 65 percent of people over age 85 are admitted to nursing homes

4.
The rationale for encouraging elders to participate in the Meals on Wheels program is to:
A. Prevent illness
B. Prolong healing
C. Prevent blindness
D. Lessen loneliness

5.

A major predictor of health status in old age is:
A. Fear of the health care system
B. Gender
C. Attitude toward aging
D. Socioeconomic status

6.
Elders who trust their health care providers usually demonstrate which of the following behaviors?
A. They view hospitals with suspicion.
B. They prefer to use their spouses or friends for health advice.
C. They generally accept their health care providers' word as law.
D. They frequently self-medicate with over-the-counter drugs.

7.
Mr. Harold Jones, aged 82, has recently lost his wife. His daughter, with whom he is living, has become concerned because he is not eating well and frequently "forgets" to turn off the electric burner on the stove when he heats up food that she has prepared for his lunch while she is at work. Mr. Jones is able to meet his activities of daily living, although his hygiene has declined since his wife's death. Which health care setting would be MOST APPROPRIATE for Mr. Jones?
A. Home health
B. Adult day care
C. Subacute care
D. Nursing home

8.
Mrs. Consuelo Bianco, aged 68, had surgery 2 weeks ago to repair a fractured hip. She is medically stable and working with a physical therapist on rehabilitation. Her husband is in poor health and is unable to provide care for her at home. They have limited financial resources. Which health care setting would be MOST APPROPRIATE for Mrs. Bianco?
A. Home health
B. Adult day care
C. Ambulatory care
D. Nursing home

Chapter 2

1.
The shift of elder care from home and family to nursing homes in the 1930s was facilitated by welfare reforms and
A. The Omnibus Budget Reconciliation Act (OBRA) of 1987
B. The American Association of Retired People (AARP)
C. Social Security
D. Medicare

2.
Concerns about the quality and availability of health care for the elderly led Congress in the 1960s to pass legislation popularly called:
A. Medicare and Medicaid
B. Social Security and unemployment insurance
C. Blue Cross and Blue Shield
D. OBRA and COBRA

3.
Mrs. Alice Smith, aged 75, is widowed and does not wish to live with either of her adult children or their families. She is physically active and enjoys her volunteer work at the local hospital. Her husband's insurance has left her financially secure. She is tired of trying to maintain her single-family house. Mrs. Smith might be MOST interested in:
A. A subacute care facility
B. An extended care facility
C. A residential care home
D. A life care retirement community

4.
Mr. Jack Higgins, aged 33, has left-sided paralysis and impaired memory following a motorcycle accident. He also has two to three seizures a day despite medication. His family is unable to provide the care that he needs and is seeking a long term care site. Mr. Higgins's needs might be best met by a nursing home with a
A. Subacute unit
B. Head injury unit
C. Respite unit
D. Dementia unit

5.
Mrs. Lettie Slaughter, aged 76, is becoming increasingly confused. She lives with her daughter who must work during the day. Mrs. Slaughter became very agitated and anxious when she went to the adult day care center and refused to

return. What health care setting could the nurse suggest to her daughter?
A. Home with a care aide
B. Respite unit
C. Dementia unit
D. Skilled nursing home

6.
What characteristics would a nurse use to describe the typical nursing home resident?
A. An under age 80, married, white man
B. An under age 65, single, white man
C. An over age 80, married, African-American woman
D. An over age 80, widowed, woman

7.
The nurse at the local nursing home has received information that a hospital client is being transferred to the nursing home for self-care instruction following surgery for a permanent colostomy. The length of stay is anticipated to be no longer than 3 weeks. The nurse would expect the new resident to be:
A. Under age 75, with few chronic illnesses, and cognitively intact.
B. Under age 75, with three or more chronic illnesses, and cognitively impaired
C. Over age 80, with no chronic illness, and cognitively intact
D. Over age 80, with several chronic illnesses, and cognitively impaired

8.
The average length of stay for a resident living in a nursing home is:
A. 6 months
B. 1 year
C. 2 years
D. 2½ years

9.
A typical chronic illness causing nursing admission for a middle-aged adult is:
A. Congestive heart failure
B. Multiple sclerosis
C. Stroke
D. Hip fracture

10.
Mrs. Betsy Watson, aged 87, was admitted to the nursing home yesterday following surgery for a fractured hip. Until her fall at home she had lived alone. Her daughter lives 3 hours away. Today Mrs. Watson is loudly screaming, "Help me, please, help me," from her wheelchair. When the nurse asks Mrs. Watson

what she needs, Mrs. Watson points a shaky finger at the wall and states, "Those snakes are coming to get me." The nurse should consider which of the following as the MOST LIKELY cause for Mrs. Watson's behavior?
A. Delusional thinking
B. Over hydration
C. Relocation syndrome
D. Sensory deprivation

11.
Mr. Marvin Donnell, aged 85, had surgery for benign prostatic hypertrophy. Following his surgery he experienced a stroke, which left him paralyzed on the left side. Mrs. Donnell is unable to care for him at home. Mr. Donnell's nurse can BEST help him make the transition to the nursing home by:
A. Referring him to the financial counselor to relieve his worries about finances
B. Talking with him about some of the experiences that he might have at the nursing home
C. Making sure that Mrs. Donnell can go with him in the ambulance
D. Making sure that the interagency transfer form is completed accurately

12.
Miss Alvira Bates, aged 92, was hospitalized 4 days ago for complications of her diabetes mellitus. She is unable to return to her home and will need nursing home placement. She is concerned about finances. The nurse should know that:
A. Medicare is available only after all personal funds have been depleted
B. Medicaid (Medical Assistance) will pay 100 percent of the cost of skilled nursing home placement
C. Medicare will pay for up to 100 days of skilled care after an initial 3-day hospital admission
D. Medicaid will pay for up to 85 percent for 100 days of skilled care after an initial 3-day hospital admission

13.
The OBRA was passed in 1987 to address quality-of-care issues in nursing homes. The survey process mandated by OBRA focuses primarily on:
A. Resident outcomes
B. Building inspection
C. Health department inspection
D. Paperwork review

14.
Voluntary accreditation is usually granted after a nursing home requests and is surveyed by the
A. American Association of Nursing Homes

B. American Healthcare Association
C. Long-Term Care Commission
D. Joint Commission on Accreditation of Healthcare Organizations

Chapter 3

1.
During a routine physical examination, Mr. Merle Bishop, aged 75, expresses concern that he must stop and rest more frequently when he is mowing the grass and that his heart pounds for "a long while" after exercise. It would be MOST IMPORTANT for the nurse to:
A. Report the finding to the physician immediately
B. Document his statements
C. Check his resting pulse rate
D. Explain the consequences of age-related changes to his heart

2.
Mrs. Nora Steary, aged 86, staggered slightly after she stood up in the doctor's office. In addition to questioning her about dizziness and faintness, the nurse would want to check her
A. Pulse rate
B. Respiratory rate
C. Blood pressure
D. Laboratory values

3.
Which of the following statements is TRUE about the effects of age-related changes on activity tolerance?
A. Changes in the cardiovascular system will cause a lower-than-normal heart rate.
B. Changes in the respiratory system will cause shortness of breath with prolonged activity.
C. Changes in the musculoskeletal system will prohibit rapid walking.
D. Changes in the renal system will increase the need for sodium replacement.

4.
Mr. Homer White, aged 78, has recently had pneumonia. Which of the following information from his medical history would alert the nurse to an increased risk of a repeated respiratory infection?
A. Dry skin with poor turgor
B. Vigorous cough reflex
C. Respiratory rate of 20/min
D. Weight gain of 0.5 pounds in 3 weeks

5.
The nurse is planning to teach Mrs. Hilda Gallagher, aged 79, diabetic self-care.

It would be MOST IMPORTANT for the nurse to structure the teaching so that:
A. All the information is in writing
B. Teaching sessions are frequent, short, and have practice time included
C. A videotape overview, which contains all the elements to be learned, is shown first
D. Mrs. Gallagher is in group of other clients who need to learn self-care

6.
Mr. Al Smith, aged 67, complains to the nurse that although he gets 6 hours of sleep a night, he never seems to feel rested. The nurse should explain that Mr. Smith probably:
A. Needs more than 6 hours of sleep
B. Needs more physical activity during the day
C. Should drink less coffee during the day
D. Has decreased REM sleep, which is normal

7.
Mrs. Adelia Robinson a 65-year-old African-American woman asks her nurse about the possibility that she might develop osteoporosis. The nurse should respond:
A. "Osteoporosis is a reversible process once diagnosed, so you needn't be concerned."
B. "Men generally have as much of a problem with osteoporosis as women, but the literature has focused more on women."
C. "Elbows and ankles are most affected by osteoporosis, but other joints may also be affected."
D. "African-American women have more bone stock than other racial groups, so they have a lower incidence of osteoporosis."

8.
At 0630, the geriatric nursing assistant (GNA) reports to the nurse that 91-year-old Mrs. Bonita Garcia's temperature is 96.2 degrees Fahrenheit. Mrs. Garcia is wearing a nightgown, has two blankets covering her, and the room temperature is 74 degrees Fahrenheit. The BEST explanation for Mrs. Garcia's temperature is:
A. The thermometer is inaccurate
B. The loss of subcutaneous tissue
C. Her nightgown is not heavy enough
D. The room temperature is too low

9.
The nurse observes Mr. George Simmons, aged 77, sitting in the day room of the nursing home with a large wet stain on his trousers over his crotch. Mr.

Simmons states, "I don't know what the problem is. I urinate and then I just somehow seem to dribble all the time." The BEST explanation for Mr. Simmons's wet spot is:
A. Stress incontinence
B. Urinary frequency
C. Benign prostatic hypertrophy
D. Decreased glomerular filtration rate

10.
Mr. Julio Martinez, aged 87, has a slightly decreased red blood cell count. He does not have any other clinically significant physical findings. The BEST explanation for his decreased red blood cell count is:
A. He is slightly dehydrated
B. His lower androgen production
C. His diet is deficient in iron
D. He has an undetected active loss of red blood cells

11.
Handwashing is especially important in the nursing home because:
A. There are more pathogens in the environment
B. Pathogens in the environment are more resistant to antibiotic therapy
C. The immune system of elders tends to function less effectively
D. Elders tend to have a higher white blood cell count

12.
Mrs. Karla Stout, aged 85, has dry, flaky skin, coarse hair, and is very slow moving. She has recently complained of feeling unable to get warm enough. She has gained approximately 15 pounds in the last year. The nurse should review her laboratory studies for:
A. Thyroid hormones
B. Adrenal hormones
C. Serum potassium concentration
D. Serum sodium concentration

13.
Mr. Saul Rosen, aged 87, has a blood urea nitrogen (BUN) level of 42 mg/dL. His daughter expresses concern that his kidneys are not functioning properly. The nurse knows:
A. A BUN level greater than 35 usually means that there is some problem with the kidneys
B. The BUN level is an accurate measure of kidney functioning
C. It is possible for elders with adequate kidney function to have a BUN level as high as 67 mg/dL

D. The BUN is a reflection of decreased protein metabolism

14.
The nurse is planning to administer medications to Mrs. Rose Hidenburg, aged 82. A review of Mrs. Hidenburg's laboratory values indicate that her hemoglobin level is 11 g/dL, her serum potassium concentration is 3.5 mEq/L, her BUN level is 37 mg/dL, and her creatinine clearance is 65 mL/min. Which of the laboratory values should concern the nurse MOST?
A. Hemoglobin level
B. Potassium concentration
C. BUN level
D. Creatinine clearance

15.
Mr. Rubin Rosenburg, aged 65, retired 6 months ago. During a routine physical examination his health care provider notices that he appears pale, listless, and answers questions very slowly. When questioned about how he is feeling, Mr. Rosenburg states, "I don't know. Nothing seems to make much sense anymore. Some days I just stay in bed." The health care provider should assess Mr. Rosenburg further for:
A. Depression
B. Iron deficiency anemia
C. Immune system dysfunction
D. Delusional thinking

16.
Mrs. Carmelita Rodriquez, aged 79, has been attending religious service at her church with her daughter every Sunday. The nurse reminds the GNA to have Mrs. Rodriquez dressed and ready to leave with her daughter. The nurse is aware that:
A. Most elders view church solely as a social event
B. Healthy elders go to church once a week
C. There is a strong association between religion and well-being
D. Although religion is comforting, it is of limited help during stressful events

17.
Ms. Ida Boyd, aged 34, is admitted to the nursing home with multiple sclerosis. She expresses concern during the admission interview that she does not see anyone her age and is uneasy. The nurse's BEST response is:
A. "We do have one resident about your age or a little older. I'll arrange a visit."
B. "Don't worry. Our social events are a lot of fun for everyone, regardless of their age."
C. "Am I correct that you are feeling uneasy? Tell me more about how you are

feeling."
D. "I'm sure you'll feel better once you get settled in. I know this is a big move for you."

18.
The preadmission screening/annual resident review (PASARR) documents screen for:
A. Financial status
B. Mental illness or mental retardation
C. Complete history and physical assessment
D. Rehabilitative potential

19.
The nursing assessment database for newly residents must be completed within 24 hours. It is the responsibility of the LPN/LVN to:
A. Gather and record information as directed by agency policy
B. Complete and sign the form
C. Delegate to the GNA the task of gathering information such as weight and height
D. Ensure the accuracy of the database by placing it in the resident's record

20.
The minimum data set (MDS) and resident assessment protocols (RAPs) can BEST be described as:
A. A comprehensive plan of care
B. A summary of medical needs of the resident
C. A list of resident goals for rehabilitation
D. An interdisciplinary assessment tool

21.
Assessment of residents in a nursing home differ from the shift-to-shift assessments of patients in acute care settings in which way?
A. Every resident is assessed by the nurse at least once every 24 hours.
B. Every resident is assessed by the interdisciplinary team every 2 weeks.
C. Physical assessments on all residents may not be done by the nurse every day.
D. Physical assessments are scheduled at least once a month.

Chapter 4

1.
Mr. Fred Ames, aged 64, has diabetic neuropathy in his legs and feet. In addition to an increased risk for infection, Mr. Ames is also at risk for:
A. Confusion
B. Deep venous thrombosis
C. Falls
D. Bunions

2.
Mr. James Startt, aged 76, has Parkinson's disease. He walks using a walker and with a slow shuffling gait. The nurse should consider him at high risk for falls because of his
A. "Pill-rolling" tremor
B. Compromised ability to move
C. Ability to use a walker
D. Mental status

3.
The nurse is assessing a newly admitted resident for fall potential. Which finding would alert the nurse to an increased risk for falls?
A. Increased BUN level
B. Decreased cardiac output
C. Decreased muscle mass
D. Cataracts

4.
Mr. Hans Holvig, aged 76, has been admitted to the nursing home from his home. His admission database indicates that he has glaucoma, benign prostatic hypertrophy, diabetes mellitus, and an acute flare-up of psoriasis. Which finding does NOT increase Mr. Holvig's fall risk?
A. Glaucoma
B. Benign prostatic hypertrophy
C. Diabetes mellitus
D. Psoriasis

5.
The nurse is administering the morning medications to assigned residents. Which observation made while she administers medications would necessitate stopping to correct the situation before continuing with medication administration?

A. A pencil on the floor
B. Two geriatric nursing assistants (GNAs) transferring a heavy resident from bed to a bath chair
C. A multilevel cart filled with water pitchers left next to the entrance to the unit kitchen
D. A laundry aide pulling a clothes rack with residents' clean laundry down the hall

6.
The nursing staff wants to implement a program to decrease the number of resident falls in the facility. What data should the staff gather FIRST?
A. Number of residents with significantly impaired mobility
B. Number of residents with significantly altered cognition
C. Time and location of falls over the past year
D. Number of staff per shift

7.
Interventions to prevent resident falls includes all the following EXCEPT:
A. Sturdy, leather-soled shoes
B. Toileting regimen of every 6 to 8 hours
C. Instruction on how to use the call bell
D. Review of medications for adverse effect

8.
The GNA has just reported that a resident has fallen in the dining room. The nurse should begin an assessment of the resident with:
A. A full head-to-toe physical assessment
B. Vital signs
C. Determination of the level of consciousness (LOC)
D. The ABCs (airway, breathing, circulation)

9.
In addition to checking vital signs and LOC, it would be MOST IMPORTANT for the nurse to evaluate a resident who has just fallen for:
A. Hyperventilation
B. A fractured hip
C. Blurred vision
D. Skin tears

10.
Mrs. Li Tranh, aged 73, fell in her bathroom. She is alert, oriented to place and time, and is able to answer questions. She complains of pain in her left groin, but there is no obvious external rotation or shortening of her left leg. The BEST

63

course of action for the nurse to take is to:
A. Document the physical findings carefully
B. Call the physician immediately to report the complaint of groin pain
C. Monitor Mrs. Tranh's activity level carefully for the rest of the shift
D. Make sure the oncoming shift is informed of Mrs. Tranh's fall

11.
The nurse is assessing a newly admitted resident for the potential for developing pressure ulcers. Which finding would alert the nurse to an increased risk for pressure ulcers?
A. Weight greater than 20 percent under ideal body weight
B. Decreased cardiac output
C. Decreased respiratory muscle elasticity
D. Unsteady gait

12.
Mrs. Hazel White, aged 63, has a history of paranoid behavior. Today Mrs. White is agitated and striking out at other residents who happen to walk near her wheelchair. She has a PRN order for haloperidol (Haldol) 1 mg PO every 6 hours for disruptive behavior. The nurse knows that giving the haloperidol will increase Mrs. White's risk for falls and
A. Visual hallucinations
B. Auditory hallucinations
C. Pressure ulcers
D. Urinary incontinence

13.
The nurse has assessed a newly admitted resident's risk for developing pressure ulcers using the Braden Scale for Predicting Pressure Sore Risk. The resident's score is 6. The nurse classifies the client's risk for pressure ulcers as:
A. Low
B. Moderate
C. High
D. Unable to be classified from the data given

14.
The GNA asks the nurse to observe a resident's right heel because the GNA is concerned that a pressure ulcer is developing. The heel is reddened, blanches when finger pressure is applied, and the skin is intact. The skin returns to pink in less than minute. The nurse should tell the nursing assistant which of the following?
A. "The heel is not at stage I yet, but be sure to keep pressure off the heel."
B. "The heel is certainly at stage I, and we will start our skin protocol now."
C. "The heel is at stage II. Start the skin protocol. I'll check it later today."
D. "The heel is at stage III. Start the skin protocol. I'll call the physician and report the problem."

15.
Mr. Sam Meadows, aged 77, is an African-American man who was admitted with left hemiparesis following a stroke from to hypertension. Mr. Meadows's GNA asks the nurse to look at his buttocks to determine if a pressure ulcer has developed. Which information makes assessment for stage I pressure ulcers more difficult for Mr. Meadows?
A. His age
B. His medical diagnosis
C. The location of the potential problem
D. The color of his skin

16.
Mrs. Magdalen Martin, aged 88, is 5 feet 7 inches tall and weighs 105 pounds. She has had a stroke, has right hemiparesis, and is incontinent. She was admitted from home because her family could not care for the pressure ulcer on her coccyx. The pressure ulcer is 5 cm wide, 3 cm long, foul-smelling and covered with black eschar. Which information makes assessment for staging Mrs. Martin's pressure ulcer more difficult?
A. Wound drainage
B. Eschar
C. Incontinence
D. Weight greater than 20 percent under ideal body weight

17.
The nurse is about to observe a resident's stage III pressure ulcer. The resident was admitted 6 days ago from an acute care facility with the pressure ulcer. The resident has foul-smelling drainage from the wound. Using the red-yellow-black system for wound classification, the nurse will expect to see:
A. Skin reddened and swollen
B. A red wound
C. A yellow wound

D. A African-American wound

18.
Mr. Donald Suitland, aged 89, has a stage III, profusely draining pressure ulcer on his left hip. The nurse would expect the wound to be treated with a regimen of cleaning the wound with an antibacterial solution and applying a
A. Hydrophilic dressing
B. Hydrophobic dressing
C. Continuous dry sterile dressing
D. Wet-to-dry dressing

19.
Mrs. Esther Wheeler, aged 65, weighs greater than 20 percent over her ideal body weight. She has a history of several abdominal surgeries and had nine pregnancies with 11 live births. She complains of "dribbling" urine when she sneezes or coughs suddenly and states that she has restricted her social activities because she can't always predict when her incontinence will occur. Mrs. Wheeler has which type of incontinence?
A. Acute
B. Stress
C. Overflow
D. Urge

20.
General measures to prevent incontinence include which of the following interventions?
A. Limit fluid intake to 1000 mL/day
B. Toilet resident every 6 to 8 hours
C. Encourage the resident to eat soft, cooked foods
D. Place the resident on a bowel regimen

21.
Prevention strategies for stress incontinence include which of the following interventions?
A. Teach the resident Kegel exercises
B. Treat and remove the cause of the problem
C. Avoid anticholinergic drugs
D. Use the Crede maneuver

22.
Prevention strategies for functional incontinence include which of the following interventions?
A. Teach the resident Kegel exercises

B. Use alpha-adrenergic medication to help retain urine
C. Toilet the resident every 1 to 2 hours
D. Use the Crede maneuver on a schedule

23.
Mrs. Hannah Gladshaw, aged 83, was admitted to the nursing home yesterday from the hospital. Following emergency gallbladder surgery, Mrs. Gladshaw became acutely agitated and combative. She was unable to return to her home. Which of the following events probably did NOT add to Mrs. Gladshaw's cognitive problems?
A. Sudden acute health problem
B. Anesthesia
C. Relocation
D. Adequate fluid intake

24.
Mr. Crawford Little, aged 73, has refused to go to the dining room to eat meals. He prefers to stay in bed with the bedcovers over his face. He has been consuming less than 50 percent of his meals. During an assessment, the nurse determines that he is unable to count backward from 100 subtracting 7 for each interval. He reports difficulty sleeping. The nurse should suspect that Mr. Little has:
A. Dementia
B. Delirium
C. Depression
D. Alzheimer's disease

25.
Mr. Leon Ewing, aged 56, has had several strokes. He has become progressively more impaired. He frequently screams for no apparent reason, and he is unable to state his name or where he is. He cannot describe what he had for his last meal nor the name of any of his family members. Mr. Ewing MOST LIKELY has:
A. Multi-infarct dementia
B. Delirium
C. Depression
D. Alzheimer's disease

26.
Interventions for the management of residents with dementia include:
A. Employing frequent changes of routine
B. Avoiding behavior triggers
C. Placing residents in high traffic areas where they are visible.

D. Adding light and background noise to stimulate memory.

27.
Mrs. Margaret Timmons, aged 78, has Alzheimer's disease. She wanders the hallways at night and frequently disturbs other residents. Mrs. Timmon's nurse implements which of the following strategies to protect the privacy of other residents?
A. Do not argue with Mrs. Timmons
B. Use gentle touch
C. Increase lighting
D. Place a large NO sign on the doors where she is not to enter

28.
Mrs. Viola Farrington, aged 85, frequently screams and strikes out when anyone approaches her wheelchair. Her nurse should plan to:
A. Reduce stimulation in her environment by placing her in a quiet location
B. Provide her with opportunities for excercise, such as dancing
C. Distract her with food or a quiet activity
D. Toilet her frequently

29.
Mr. Charles Holmes, aged 67, has progressive dementia and has been identified as having a high risk for falls after two actual falls. The LEAST preferred intervention for reducing Mr. Holmes's fall risk when he is sitting in a chair is a
A. "Lap Buddy"
B. Wedge pillow
C. Waist restraint
D. Reclining chair

30.
Based on a review of the daily food intake record, a nurse suspects that a resident is not receiving adequate nutrition. Which of the following laboratory studies would provide early confirmation that the resident has inadequate nutrition?
A. A weight loss of 3 pounds over 5 weeks
B. A low thyroxine PAB level
C. A body mass index of 23
D. A low serum albumin concentration

31.
Mr. Harold Wong, aged 74, was admitted to the nursing home 6 months ago. His primary diagnosis was severe congestive heart failure. He also has cataracts, hearing loss, and has fallen several times. A monthly review of Mr. Wong's

chart reveals that he has had a weight loss of 6.5 pounds. The nurse's first action is to:
A. Review his medications for diuretic therapy
B. Ask the GNA to reweigh him
C. Plan to reweigh him at the same time of day next week to see whether the weight loss continues
D. Note the loss and make sure his physician is notified.

32.
Mrs. Hannah Goldstein, aged 67, has had a stroke and has been treated for a poorly healing pressure ulcer on her coccyx. Her nurse notes that Mrs. Goldstein has had several urinary tract infections and colds in the past 8 months. A review of her laboratory tests shows that her red blood cell count is low normal, white blood cell count is low normal, her serum albumin concentration is low, and her serum cholesterol level is low. The nurse should suspect that Mrs. Goldstein has:
A. An active infection
B. A high risk for falls
C. Liver disease
D. Malnutrition

33.
Mr. Julio Vasquez, aged 69, was admitted to the nursing home from the hospital where he had an above-the-knee amputation of his left leg from the complications of diabetes mellitus. He also has chronic renal failure and is blind. Mr. Vasquez frequently told his family, the nurses, and his physician that he did not wish to be kept alive with "tubes and machines" if his condition should decline. His admission form contained a signed statement that he did not want a feeding tube. Mr. Vasquez suffered a massive cerebral vascular hemorrhage and is comatose. The GNA assigned to his care asks why he does not have a feeding tube. The nurse's BEST response is:
A. "Well, it won't do any good, and it will just cost his family a great deal of money."
B. "His family feels that it will just prolong his misery."
C. "Mr. Vasquez was very clear that he did not want a feeding tube. We are following his directive."
D. "I know that it seems cruel, but a terminally ill person really does better without food or fluids."

34.
The risk of aspiration of enteral nutrition is decreased with the use of a
A. Nasogastric tube
B. Nasoduodenal tube

C. Nasoenteral tube
D. Gastrostomy tube

35.
Mrs. Rosa Loren, aged 78, had a percutaneous endoscopic gastrostomy (PEG) tube inserted 24 hours ago. Before the nurse begins Mrs. Loren's first tube feeding, the nurse should FIRST:
A. Check for an x-ray report that the PEG tube was placed correctly
B. Check the enteral feeding order to be sure that the correct strength is charged to Mrs. Loren.
C. Aspirate gastric contents from the tube and check the pH
D. Make sure that there is a enteral feeding flow control pump available

36.
Complications associated with tube feedings include all the following EXCEPT:
A. Aspiration pneumonia
B. Clogging
C. Impaired mobility
D. Diarrhea

37.
A resident with normal eating patterns has a distended abdomen and complains of discomfort. A review of the resident's bowel sheet over the past 4 days indicates that the resident has not had a bowel movement. The nurse's FIRST action should be:
A. A review of the resident's food consumption for the past week
B. Light palpation of the entire abdomen
C. Auscultation of abdomen in all four quadrants
D. A digital rectal examination to palpate for an impaction

38.
Prevention interventions for constipation include:
A. Recording the resident's bowel movements
B. Establishing a bowel routine
C. Limiting visitors until bowel function returns to normal
D. Disimpacting the bowel

39.
Mrs. Maria Donatello, aged 69, has had several large watery stools today. Which of the following information gathered from her chart might indicate why she has the diarrhea?
A. She has eaten 100 percent of her meals for the past 10 days.
B. She has had antibiotic therapy for a urinary tract infection.

C. She has eaten in the dining room at a table with other residents.
D. She has consumed 1500 mL of water every day.

40.
When planning care for a resident with diarrhea, the MOST IMPORTANT intervention is:
A. Antidiarrheal agents
B. Anti-infective agents for the causative agent, if the diarrhea is from infection
C. Isolation
D. Fluid administration to prevent dehydration

Chapter Five

1.
The rationale for encouraging elders to get all their prescription and over-the-counter drugs from the same pharmacy is:
A. The drugs will cost less in the long run
B. A complete record of all medications permits the pharmacist to check for drug interactions
C. The health care provider can give better instructions for filling the prescription
D. Elders are less apt to forget where they got the prescription filled

2.
An elder at high risk for polypharmacy would demonstrate a
A. Low incidence of chronic illness
B. Low number of side effects from prescribed medications
C. Knowledgeable health care provider
D. Tendency to self-medicate for minor problems

3.
Which of the following is a health care provider action that increases the risk of polypharmacy in elderly clients ?
A. Frequent continuing education on drug therapy for information on newest treatment protocols
B. Leaving residents on the same medications for extended periods of time, adding drugs as needed for acute problems
C. Frequent reviews of pharmaceutical protocols for adjustments
D. Regularly ordering lower than stated normal doses for elders with liver or kidney problems

4.
Mrs. Mary Stankowitz, aged 85, is 5 feet 3 inches tall and weighs 87 pounds. She is diabetic, has peptic ulcer disease (PUD), and has had a stroke but is able to walk with a walker. Mrs. Stankowitz is at risk for poor drug absorption of insulin because:
A. Most forms of insulin will cause her PUD to flare-up
B. Her mobility is slowed with her walker when she walks daily
C. She probably has inadequate subcutaneous tissue.
D. She has malabsorption syndrome

5.
Mr. Dan Marvelle, 76, is receiving verapamil (Calan), furosemide (Lasix), and

digoxin. A review of Mr. Marvelle's laboratory studies reveals the following test results: hematocrit 45%, BUN 35, serum potassium 4.0 mEq/L, and serum albumin 2.8 g/L. Which of the test values should concern the nurse?
A. Hematocrit level
B. BUN level
C. Serum potassium concentration
D. Serum albumin concentration

6.
Mr. Grigori Stanka, aged 64, has hypertension and is post-stroke status. He is receiving digoxin, furosemide (Lasix), and phenytoin (Dilantin) for his medical problems. His medical history also includes information that Mr. Stanka drank a pint to a quart of vodka a day for 25 to 30 years. Mr. Stanka's nurse should observe him especially carefully for:
A. Toxic side effects of his medication
B. Skin breakdown from his impaired mobility
C. Changes in his mental status
D. Depression

7.
The primary strategy to prevent complications of drug therapy is to:
A. Make sure residents take their medications as ordered by their health care provider
B. "Start low, go slow"
C. "Start high, go low"
D. Rapidly increase drug doses until therapeutic effects are achieved

8.
Mrs. Hannah Goldbaum, aged 77, has been given ibuprofen (Motrin) 400 mg PO every 6 hours for joint pain as ordered by her health care provider. Which of Mrs. Goldbaum's statements to the nurse would indicate that the ibuprofen should be withheld until her health care provider can be notified?
A. "I feel sleepy all the time even though I get lots of sleep."
B. "I get lightheaded when I get up suddenly."
C. "My mouth seems dry all the time."
D. "I had a lot of blood on my toothbrush this morning."

9.
One of reasons why elders have frequently been under medicated for pain is that nurses:
A. Have been taught to accurately assess a resident's pain level
B. Accurately distinguish among the types of pain
C. Recommend appropriate nonpharmacological interventions for pain control

measures
D. Are concerned about sedation and respiratory depression with elders

10.
The nurse working with an elder on pain control would want to include which of the following facts in a teaching plan?
A. Narcotics should be avoided because they are addictive
B. Mild pain is common and should not require medication
C. Reassure the resident that they are not "a bother" if they request pain medication.
D. Moderate to severe pain indicates impending death.

11.
Mr. Marvin Schwartz, aged 66, has had severe peripheral vascular disease for nearly 10 years. He had an above-the-knee amputation of his right leg 2 years ago. He admits to constant pain in his left leg when questioned. Which of the following behaviors by Mr. Schwartz would indicate that his pain is not being well controlled?
A. Elevated pulse and blood pressure
B. Restlessness
C. Depression
D. Sweating

12.
The nurse assessing a confused resident for pain should plan to use which of the following assessment strategies?
A. The P-Q-R-S-T model
B. Observations for grimacing or guarding
C. A linear pain scale
D. An interview with the resident's physician

13.
Mrs. Sally Martin, aged 69, was admitted to the nursing home 10 hours ago from the hospital. She had surgery 6 days ago to repair a fractured hip. She received a dose of morphine at the hospital just before she was transferred and has received two doses of acetaminophen 500 mg PO since admission to the nursing home. At this time she is crying and states that her hip "is aching like a toothache" and rates her pain as 9 on a scale of 0 to 10. She wants mediation for pain. Her medical orders say that the acetaminophen is to be given every 4 to 6 hours, and her last dose was 3 hours ago. The nurse should:
A. Give her another dose of acetaminophen
B. Try distraction and guided imagery
C. Move her leg and give her a backrub

D. Call her physician and report Mrs. Martin's pain

14.
Mr. Robert Butler, aged 88, has a history of congestive heart failure and angina. He has been nauseated and vomiting for 2 days. His physician orders an intravenous infusion to maintain his hydration. The nurse would question which of the following infusion therapy orders?
A. 1000-mL 0.9 percent saline IV at 30 mL/hr
B. 1000-mL 5 percent D/W IV at 30 mL/hr
C. 1000-mL 5 percent D/0, 45 percent saline IV at 100 mL/hr
D. 1000-mL 5 percent D/W IV at 50 mL/hr

15.
Mr. Andy Williams, aged 63, has metastatic colon cancer. He is on a regimen of peripheral parenteral nutrition (PPN). Which of the following assessment findings should alert the nurse to a major complication of PPN?
A. Temperature of 101 degrees Fahrenheit
B. Complaints of abdominal pain
C. Bleeding gums
D. Weight loss of 0.25 pounds in 3 weeks

Chapter Six

1.
Many factors predispose the elderly to acute infections. Which of the following factors is MOST LIKELY to add to the risk of infection?
A. A balanced 1500-calorie diet for a bedridden resident
B. A fluid intake of 1900 mL per 24 hours for a resident
C. Crowded living quarters and many visitors
D. Yearly flu shots

2.
Of all the infection control strategies, which of the following is MOST IMPORTANT for prevention of acute infection in the elderly?
A. Handwashing
B. Placing residents in a 45-degree upright position for 1 hour after tube feeding
C. Receiving annual immunizations for influenza
D. Assuring a fluid intake of 2000 mL per 24 hours on residents who are not fluid restricted

3.
Mr. George McCloud, aged 76, has non–insulin-dependent diabetes mellitus (NIDDM) and is able to meet his normal daily needs. His medical history also indicates that he has benign prostatic hypertrophy. In planning care to prevent infection, it would be MOST IMPORTANT for the nurse to include which of the following interventions for Mr. McCloud?
A. Turn, cough, and deep breathe every 2 hours
B. Inspect the urine frequently for color, clarity, and odor
C. Encourage the resident to eat a 1600-calorie American Diabetes Association diet
D. Encourage the resident to take annual immunization shots

4.
Which of the following assessment data would indicate a likely fluid volume deficit?
A. Increased pulse rate
B. Increased respiratory rate
C. Increased body temperature
D. Pale, clammy skin

5.
Which of the following assessment data would indicate a likely fluid volume

overload?
A. Decreased blood pressure
B. Dark, concentrated urine
C. Decreased pulse rate
D. Crackles in the lung bases

6.
The nurse should anticipate which of the following interventions for an elderly resident with a fluid volume defict?
A. Placing the head of the bed in a high semi-Fowler position
B. Oral replacement therapy
C. Diuretic therapy
D. Angiotensin-converting enzyme inhibitor therapy

7.
The nurse should anticipate which of the following interventions for an elderly resident with a fluid volume overload?
A. Oxygen therapy
B. Frequent mouth care
C. Assistance when changing positions to prevent falls
D. Daily application of body lotion

8.
Ms. Alvira Bates, aged 64, has congestive heart failure and has been taking a loop diuretic in addition to other medications. Yesterday, she complained of nausea and fatigue. The geriatric nursing assistant (GNA) reported that Ms. Bates had two watery stools and vomited once between 0700 and 1200. The nurse's assessment revealed that Mrs. Bates is now very weak and has a very irregular heartbeat. The nurse should suspect that Ms. Bates has a
A. Sodium excess
B. Sodium deficit
C. Potassium excess
D. Potassium deficit

9.
The nurse caring for a resident with a low serum potassium level should question a medication order for:
A. Calcium carbonate
B. Furosemide (Lasix)
C. Levothyronine (Synthroid)
D. Lisinopril (Zestril)

10.

Mr. Alberto Gomez, aged 75, has been treated for congestive heart failure with diet and fluid restrictions and a loop diuretic in addition to other medications. The GNA has reported that Mr. Gomez is far more confused this morning than usual. A nursing assessment reveals that Mr. Gomez is lethargic, confused, and is unable to state where he is or the day. The nurse should suspect that Mr. Gomez has a:
A. Sodium excess
B. Sodium deficit
C. Potassium excess
D. Potassium deficit

11.
Ms. Debra Polevoy, aged 62, has congestive heart failure, insulin-dependent diabetes mellitus and a history of urinary tract infections. The GNA reports that Ms. Polevoy is complaining of weakness and fatigue this morning. A nursing assessment reveals that Ms. Polevoy has warm, dry skin; dry, sticky mucous membranes; dark, concentrated urine; and deep blowing respirations. The nurse should suspect that Ms. Polevoy has:
A. Pneumonia
B. Diabetic ketoacidosis
C. Fluid overload
D. A urinary tract infection

12.
Mr. George Siemonds, aged 72, has a history of NIDDM. He is complaining of fatigue; his skin is warm, dry and flushed; his breathing and breath are within his normal baseline; and his mucous membranes are dry and sticky. His nurse should expect to find his finger-stick blood glucose to be:
A. Less than 60 mg/dL
B. Between 60 and 120 mg/dL
C. Between 300 to 600 mg/dL
D. Greater than 600 mg/dL

13.
Mrs. Antoinette Mignonne, aged 82, awoke during the night and complained of severe indigestion. This morning, she is again complaining of indigestion unrelieved by an antacid. She also is complaining of extreme fatigue. Her nurse should suspect that Mrs. Mignonne may have which of the following conditions?
A. Angina
B. Atypical myocardial infarction
C. Pneumonia
D. Duodenal ulcer

14.
Which of the following interventions would the nurse expect to be included in the plan of care for a resident with angina?
A. Nitroglygerin by mouth every 10 minutes for a total of four tablets
B. Nitroglycerin sublingually every 5 minutes for a total of three tablets
C. Light activity until chest discomfort stops
D. Oxygen at 7 L/ min until the chest discomfort stops

15.
Which of the following assessment data indicate a deep venous thrombosis?
A. Pain is diffuse and severe.
B. The skin is pale, mottled, or cyanotic.
C. The skin over the affected area is swollen and warm.
D. Distal pulses are absent or decreased.

16. Which of the following assessment data indicate an acute arterial occlusion?
A. Mucsles are tender and indurated.
B. Pain is localized near affected area.
C. The affected area is reddened.
D. Pulses are not affected.

Chapter 7

1.
Which of the following residents would benefit MOST from the use of clinical pathways?
A. A 45-year-old single woman with advanced multiple sclerosis who needs complete care
B. A 72-year-old woman who has bilateral above-the-knee amputations and whose spouse is unable to assist her at home
C. An 84-year-old man who needs to learn to care for his ileostomy following surgery for cancer
D. A 54-year-old divorced man with post-head trauma status and unstable emotions

2.
The clinical pathway for a resident identified as high risk for impaired skin integrity. The pathway called for maintaining intact skin by turning the resident at least every 2 hours and by providing skin care three times a day. After 4 days, the resident developed a stage 2 skin lesion. The nurse noted the skin lesion on skin sheet of the resident's chart. The nurse made a further note that described the plan of care and the results but did not include the note on the resident's chart. The further note was:
A. Quality improvement documentation
B. Variance documentation
C. Alterations in the comprehensive plan of care
D. A record for personal information

3.
When documenting on the resident's progress note it would be important for the nurse to:
A. Make sure that the date and time are on each entry, as well as the writer's name and title
B. Leave plenty of white space so that someone else can write in
C. Use vague terminology or labels such as "normal day" or "cooperative"
D. Use appears or apparently rather than definite descriptions

4.
Purposes for documenting resident progress include all of the following EXCEPT:
A. Meeting requirements for financial reimbursement
B. Documenting adequate assessment

C. Making sure that residents or their families have no basis for a lawsui.
D. Communicating with other health team members

5.
The following nurses' notes are examples of which method of charting a resident's progress?
"0700 Resident up to bathroom, dressed, and walked to dining room for breakfast. No complaints of hip pain." _____N. Nurse, LPN
"1750 Visitors in to see resident. Resident smiling and talkative." _____S. Smith, RN
"2330 Resident appears to be sleeping quietly." _____M. Jones, LPN
A. Narrative charting
B. PIE charting
C. Focus charting
D. Variance charting

6.
One disadvantage of focus charting is that:
A. All phases of the nursing process are recorded as part of the note
B. It may contain needless or meaningless information
C. It uses more space on the paper
D. It may be difficult to find information easily

7.
A nurse completes an ordered antibiotic dressing on a resident's skin tear. In addition to noting improvement in the extent of the skin tear on the skin assessment record, on what other documentation record will the nurse need to record information?
A. Incident report
B. Medication administration record
C. Variance report
D. Daily activity sheet

8.
Which of the following statements about an incident report is CORRECT?
A. An incident report is used to record routine occurrences.
B. It is not necessary for the information on the nurse's note in the resident's chart to match the information on the incident report.
C. The incident report should indicate who was at fault for an occurrence.
D. Incident reports should be kept separate from the resident's record in a secure area.

Chapter Eight

1.
The relationship between health promotion and health protection can BEST be described as:
A. Health protection is a subactivity of health promotion
B. Health promotion is a subactivity of health protection
C. Health promotion is concerned with illness prevention only
D. Health protection is concerned with various activities that enhance wellness

2.
Mrs. Mary Begay, aged 67, has been admitted to the nursing home for intensive physical therapy following a total hip replacement. Her nurse is concerned that Mrs. Begay is an insulin-dependant diabetic who is greater than 20 percent over ideal body weight and who admits that she does not routinely check her blood sugar. In planning care for Mrs. Begay, comprehensive health protection instruction should focus on:
A. Diet instruction
B. Weight reduction
C. All aspects of diabetes management
D. Health benefits of a walking regimen

3.
Which of the following trends among long term care residents makes a shift to health promotion imperative?
A. Extended lengths of stay in long term care facilities
B. The shorter life expectancy of long term care residents
C. The increased incidence of acute illnesses
D. The increased incidence of chronic diseases

4.
Mr. Alvie Tso, aged 78, has been admitted to a long term care facility because of increasing confusion and inability to meet his daily care needs. Which of the following nursing interventions is directed at health promotion?
A. Reorient by using large daily calendar.
B. Encourage resident to walk briskly each day.
C. Help resident comb his hair.
D. Monitor resident's bowel movements.

5.

Mr. Rafael Mendoza, aged 72, has had non–insulin-dependant diabetes mellitus (NIDDM) for 15 years. When assessing Mr. Mendoza for health promotion instruction, the nurse should:
A. Find out what Mr. Mendoza knows about his health problem
B. Review the disease pathophysiology with Mr. Mendoza
C. Provide Mr. Mendoza with written material about the diet he has been ordered
D. Plan to take his blood sugar to determine whether it has been elevated

6.
Mr. Mohammad Mustapha, aged 64, has been unsteady on his feet. The physical therapist has been teaching him how to walk with a four-point cane. In evaluating Mr. Mustapha's progress, it would be MOST IMPORTANT for Mr. Mustapha's nurse to:
A. Tell his geriatric nursing assistant (GNA) to place him in a shower chair for bathing
B. Remind him to use the siderails in the hallway when he walks
C. Make sure that he is assisted to the dining room
D. Note on his record that he is walking correctly with the four-point cane

7.
Mrs. Agatha Cress, aged 78, has been admitted to the subacute unit for supervised instruction on how to manage her Koch's pouch urinary diversion device. Her nurse notes that Mrs. Cress is frequently confused when the nurse tries to show her self-care at the scheduled dressing change time of 1400. The nurse should FIRST consider which of the following teachng strategies?
A. Make sure that the instruction is short, simple, and repeated frequently.
B. Make sure that Mrs. Cress's family is available to help with instruction.
C. Change the dressing/instruction time to early morning.
D. Make sure that all instruction is in writing.

8.
The nurse is planning a teaching session on foot care for several residents in an assisted living building with NIDDM. In addition to scheduling a quiet room, the nurse should consider which of the following strategies?
A. Music
B. Visual aides such as a foot model
C. Schedule the session for just before supper
D. No repetition of information

Chapter Nine

1.
An elderly widow is 3 days post-operative status following a total hip replacement. She will need intensive physical therapy on a daily basis. She lives alone and has a working daughter who lives 2 hours away. Which setting would BEST meet this patient's needs?
A. The hospital's orthopedic unit
B. A transitional care unit
C. A traditional nursing home
D. Home with a home health aide 4 hours daily

2.
A patient was transferred to a transitional care unit in a nursing home. Upon arrival at the facility, the patient became very agitated and cried. When questioned, the patient stated, "My family told me that I was going to a subacute care facility. This is the nursing home. They put me here just to get rid of me!" The nurse's BEST response is:
A. "I am sure that your family has your best interests at heart. They selected the best place for you to be right now."
B. "You seem to be very upset. Perhaps we should let you rest a while before continuing with the admission procedures."
C. "I can see that you are very upset. It might be helpful to you to know that nearly all subacute units are located in nursing homes like the one here."
D. "I know that all of this has been really sudden. Most of our patients felt very much the the same way when they first arrived."

3.
Maryvale Nursing Home opened a subacute (SA) unit 9 months ago. The administrator of Maryvale wishes to have Joint Commission on Accreditation of Healthcare Organization's (JCAHO) accreditation specifically for the SA unit because she feels that the community will recognize accreditation as a standard of excellence. In order to receive JCAHO accreditation as an SA unit, the SA unit must FIRST meet:
A. JCAHO standards for long-term care
B. Only federal requirements for SA units
C. Only state requirements for SA units
D. A voluntary state survey for compliance with state and federal regulations

4.
In addition to the Joint Commission on Accreditation of Healthcare

Organizations (JCAHO), SA units may seek accreditation from which of the following accrediting bodies?
A. National Association of Subacute Units
B. Commission for Accreditation of Rehabilitation Facilities
C. American Association of Skilled and Subacute Facilities
D. American Academy of Nursing Home Administrators

5.
A patient was admitted to the hospital as a result of an automobile accident, which caused severe spinal cord damage and paralysis of the lower extremities. During treatment the patient developed a stage IV pressure ulcer on the left hip. The MOST APPROPRIATE SA placement for this patient would be:
A. Transitional SA care
B. Medical-surgical SA care
C. Long term transitional SA care
D. Home with daily nurse visits for wound care

6.
A patient with amyotrophic lateral sclerosis (ALS) has become ventilator dependent. Following hospitalization for a respiratory infection, the patient might BEST be placed in a
A. Transitional SA care
B. Medical-surgical SA care
C. Long term transitional SA care
D. Home with daily visits by a nurse and respiratory therapist

7.
A nurse is applying for a position as a staff nurse on a long term transitional SA care unit that accepts ventilator-dependent residents. In addition to knowledge of general medical-surgical nursing and geriatric nursing, it would be especially important for the nurse to have which of the following experience?
A. 2 years in long term care
B. 2 years on a medical-surgical unit in an acute care setting
C. 2 years on a rehabilitation unit
D. 2 years of critical care experience

8.
Compared with the staffing levels on traditional long term care units, those on SA units are usually:
A. About the same
B. 1.5 to 2 times greater
C. 2.5 to 3 times greater
D. Not more than 3.5 times greater

9.
The role of the nurse as case manager in subacute care can best be described as:
A. Coordinating the care given by an interdisciplinary team
B. Coordinating the care given only in SA care
C. Coordinating care to focus on a limited number of measurable client outcomes
D. Coordinating care to maximize cost-benefit results

Chapter 10

1.
A nurse has accepted a position as head nurse on a traditional long term care unit in a nearby facility. During her employment interview, the director of nursing mentioned an employee stock option in the corporation that owned the nursing home. The nurse should assume that ownership of the facility is:
A. Not-for-profit privately owened
B. Not-for-profit church owned
C. Not-for-profit government owned
D. For-profit

2.
Most facilities, whether non-for-profit or for-profit, have a group of people who are responsible for the financial and operational aspects of the organization. These people are legally responsible for:
A. Ensuring that residents receive all the care they need
B. Conforming with all the state and federal regulations
C. Making sure that the mission of the organization is carried out exactly as stated
D. Using any profits wisely

3.
The primary responsibility of the nursing home administrator (NHA) is to ensure that:
A. Care is given under budgeted costs
B. Quality care is given regardless of cost
C. Care given is acceptable to meet federal, state, and local standards, regardless of cost
D. Care given is high quality and cost effective

4.
In addition to a board of directors, the NHA is accountable to the state:
A. board for nurses
B. board for NHAs
C. department of social services.
D. department of licensing

5.
The charge nurse on a long term care unit has a question regarding the dosage of a medication that the physician has ordered today for one of his patients. The

nurse should direct the question FIRST to the:
A. Physician
B. Consultant pharmacist
C. Medication nurse
D. Nursing supervisor

6.
The geriatric nursing assistant (GNA) reports that a resident has lost 5 pounds in one month. After verifying that the weight was accurate by reweighing the resident, the nurse should plan to FIRST:
A. Report the finding to the physician
B. Call the dietary department for a consult with the registered dietitian
C. Have someone sit with the resident at mealtimes to assist with feeding
D. Review the food intake records to determine whether the resident is eating all of the ordered dietitian

7.
Residents' families frequently ask what function environmental services provides for their family members. The nurse's BEST reply is:
A. "The environmental services people wash and dry both residents' and the facility's laundry and deliver clean personal laundry to the residents."
B. "They are responsible for assuring that the physical surroundings are safe and in working order and that the grounds are safe."
C. "The evironmental services personnel clean the residents' rooms and are responsible for keeping floors and public use rooms clean."
D. "They are responsible for providing clerical support, such as accounting personnel, receptionists, and secretaries."

8.
A resident's son asks the nurse about the function of a person whose name badge indicates that they are the continuous quality improvement (CQI) coordinator. The nurse should respond by saying that "The CQI coordinator
A. Reviews medical records to make recommendations for improvement"
B. Arranges for staff educational programs"
C. Surveys the physical surroundings for safety compliance"
D. Reviews the care given here and compares that care to preset industry standards"

9.
Smaller nursing homes that do not have a number of rehabilitative services available may need to call in a consultant to plan care for a resident's problem. The appropriate consultant referral for a resident who has developed swallowing difficulties is the

A. Occupational therapist
B. Speech-language pathologist
C. Physical therapist
D. Activity therapist

Chapter 11

1.
The director of nursing (DON) is responsible for budgetary aspects of the nursing department. Staff have requested that an electronic bedscale be purchased to make weighing bedfast residents easier and safer. The DON would include the scale in the:
A. Operational budget
B. Capital budget
C. Revenues
D. Expenses

2.
Among other position responsibilities, the DON can generally expect to spend several hours a week doing each of the following EXCEPT:
A. Providing direct nursing care to clients
B. Recruiting and retention of staff
C. Public relations and marketing
D. Serving as resource for staff

3.
In the future, DONs in long term care can be expected to have:
A. Less responsibility than the position now includes
B. Limited ability to communicate with an interdisciplinary team
C. At least a baccalaureate degree
D. Little input into the financial aspects of long term care

4.
The assistant director of nursing (ADON) usually is concerned with:
A. Disciplining poor work performance
B. Preparing budgets
C. Monitoring utilization review and management
D. Work schedules and staffing needs

5.
Ongoing evaluation of quality nursing care provides an important link back to which management function?
A. Planning
B. Employee selection
C. Organizational culture
D. Consumer advocacy

6.
The DON has reviewed a number of incident reports submitted by the staff. The analysis of data shows that both falls and pressure ulcers appear to be increasing in this period as compared with the same period a year ago. In addition to the nursing home administrator, the DON should take the information to the
A. Infection control committee
B. Utilization review committee
C. Risk management committee
D. Quality improvement committee

7.
Risk managment can BEST be described as:
A. Tracking and monitoring infection and preventing infection
B. Instituting measures to promote residents' safety and prevention of medical malpractice
C. Performing periodic reevaluation of the level of care required by a resident
D. Determining a clinical problem, with interventions for improvement

8.
On Unit 1, the charge nurse does the treatments for all unit residents, the geriatric medicine aide (GMA) passes the oral and topical medications, and each aide is assigned to a group of residents who will need assistance with activities of daily living. In addition, each aide is assigned to special jobs, such as weekly weights, daily blood pressures, and so forth. The nursing care delivery pattern is:
A. Functional
B. Team
C. Primary
D. Resident centered

9.
On Unit 2, a subacute unit, the nurse and several geriatric nursing assistants (GNAs) are assigned to provide total care to a group of residents. The nurse also coordinates care with the interdisciplinary team. The nursing care delivery pattern is:
A. Functional
B. Primary
C. Case method
D. Resident centered

10.
The GMA can be expected to:
A. Administer oral medications

B. Do simple dry sterile dressing changes
C. Provide direct care for residents
D. Regulate intravenous fluids

11.
The GMA can be expected to:
A. Regulate intravenous fluids
B. Administer oral and certain topical medications
C. Do simple dry sterile dressing changes
D. Regulate intravenous fluids

12.
The case manager in long term care can be expected to perform each of the following functions for assigned residents EXCEPT:
A. Collaborate with the physical therapist for an appropriate exercise regimen
B. Monitor the progress of a subacute residents' ability to manage their own colostomy care
C. Clarify residents' concerns with their physicians to improve communication about end-of-life issues
D. Impose tight bugetary constraints on resident care to improve health care costs

Chapter 12

1.
A charge nurse knows that her residents expect to participate in care decisions and believes that they have the right to make choices about their care. These beliefs are BEST reflected in which of the following actions?
A. Requiring all televisions to be shut off at 2300
B. Strictly adhering to the organization's philosophy on the residents' right to privacy
C. Strongly encouraging residents to participate in the residents' council
D. Limiting access to the unit kitchen during late evening hours

2.
Being "in charge" of a unit means:
A. The person should be an RN
B. Responsibility for the nursing staff of the unit for a set period of time
C. A full-time managerial position
D. Accountability for everything that happens on the nursing unit for a set period of time

3.
Complete change of shift reports with new personnel should consist of:
A. Brief summaries of client progress
B. Client's name, physician, admitting diagnosis, and current condition
C. Client identification, medical plans, nursing plans, and concerns that need follow-up
D. Sequenced, organized data given to all members of the oncoming shift

4.
Which of the following statements about a nursing home resident is appropriate for the change of shift report?
A. "He is a real flirt."
B. "Mr. Jones in 309A fell during the night and should be checked for bruises this morning."
C. "He says that his 'waterworks' quit on him."
D. "He is a real sweetie."

5.
When a nurse assigns tasks to a nursing assistant, is the nurse liable for whether they are done correctly?
A. Never

B. Occasionally, but not usually
C. Yes
D. Because situations vary so much, the nurse would need legal advice on each situation

6.
When assigning client care, the charge nurse needs to consider all the following EXCEPT:
A. Client needs
B. Staff number and type
C. Continuity of care
D. Cost per staff hour of care

7.
A common cause of underdelegation is:
A. Trustworthy subordinates
B. A democratic leadership style
C. A need for perfection and control
D. Inadequate time to accomplish nursing care goals

8.
Which of the following is generally an inappropriate reason for delegation?
A. Delegation empowers a subordinate by "stretching" them in their work assignment.
B. Delegation frees the charge nurse to address more complex, higher-level unit needs.
C. The task is boring and the charge nurse does not want to do it.
D. Someone is better qualified to complete the task that needs to be done.

9.
All the following are requirements for delegating duties and tasks EXCEPT:
A. Identifying the staff member to whom tasks are to be delegated
B. Determining that the work is consistent with the staff member's job description
C. Obtaining the staff member's voluntary acceptance of the work request
D. Giving direction and supervision only upon request

10.
All of the following are suggestions for developing effective delegation skills EXCEPT:
A. Clarifying the delegated tasks
B. Allowing the staff member to participate
C. Providing the staff member with the right to fully determine how and when

the job is to be done
D. Establishing feedback channels

11.
A unit coordinator assists a group of nursing personnel to resolve a conflict by defining values and goals openly, reponsibly, and in an environment of trust and committment. This approach is called:
A. Compromise
B. Capitulation
C. Collaboration
D. Accommodation

12.
The unit coordinator, Marge Grantham, is meeting with two other unit coordinators regarding the budget for next year. Each needs several pieces of expensive equipment. Mrs. Grantham, after thinking about the situation, proposes that each unit reexamine its needs and select less expensive items, and in turn, she will not submit a request for a very expensive item that her unit really needs. The strategy will allow all units to get at least part of what they need. This is an example of what type of conflict resolution?
A. Accommodating
B. Avoiding
C. Competing
D. Compromising

13.
You are in line in the facility cafeteria and have only 20 minutes for your lunch. The Minimum Data Set coordinator who has been reviewing your unit's records steps in front of you in the salad line. Rather than challenge her rudeness, you just step back. You have had a particularly hectic morning, and in addition, you are counting on a recommendation from this individual for a merit increase. This action is an example of which type of conflict resolution?
A. Accommodation
B. Avoidance
C. Competion
D. Compromise

14.
A leader who tends to involve subordinates in decision making, delegates authority, and uses participation and feedback would be described as:
A. Democratic
B. Laissez-faire
C. Authorative

D. Autocratic

15.
A leader who tends to centralize authority and limit subordinate participation would be described as:
A. Democratic
B. Laissez-faire
C. Authorative
D. Autocratic

Chapter Thirteen

1.
The purpose for a survey is BEST described as:
A. An official inspection to determine compliance with state and federal laws
B. A voluntary inspection to assure residents of high-quality care
C. An unannounced voluntary inspection of the facility by a team of surveyors
D. A scheduled official inspection of the facility by one or two surveyors

2.
The survey includes all the following elements EXCEPT that:
A. The structure of the process is predetermined
B. The findings are confidential
C. The survey is conducted by state employed surveyors
D. The survey is conducted by a team of surveyors, which usually includes a nurse

3.
As compared to the quality of care assessment, the environmental quality assessment is more concerned with evidence that:
A. Residents are enabled to reach their highest level of physical, mental, and psychosocial well-being
B. Residents' drug regimens are appropriate
C. The physical aspects of the facility's environment are safe and promote resident well-being
D. Residents' rights are being safeguarded

4.
Both the resident and the family councils can BEST be described as:
A. Official groups that meet to discuss issues related to resident care or the operation of the facility
B. Official social groups that provide support for residents and their families
C. Unofficial groups that meet whenever a resident has a complaint about the facility
D. Unofficial groups that meet regularly to determine the social activities to be offered by the facility

5.
Mrs. Smith is very concerned about her mother who is a resident of a long term care facility. Mrs. Smith has noted that one or two confused residents frequently wander into her mother's room and rummage through her belongings. Mrs.

Smith has asked that the door to her mother's room be closed at all times. The nurses have explained that having the door closed is against facility policy. Having gotten no satisfaction from the floor staff, Mrs. Smith should take her concerns to the:
A. Residents' council
B. Family council
C. Quality of life committee
D. Interdisciplinary team

6.
During a drug therapy review, a surveyor would usually NOT look at which of the following to determine that residents are being appropriately medicated?
A. The physician's order
B. The medication administration record (MAR)
C. The diet sheet
D. Laboratory studies

7.
A resident has been placed on phenytoin (Dilantin) 100 mg. orally three times a day for seizures following a cerebrovascular accident. The nurse would expect to see the reason for the drug to be clearly identified in each of the following EXCEPT:
A. Physician's orders
B. Physician's progress notes
C. MAR
D. Daily activities record

8.
A staff nurse was encouraged by the supervisor to attend the survey team's exit conference. The staff nurse should expect that the conference will:
A. Clearly identify residents whose care was found to be substandard.
B. Identify deficiencies found by the survey team
C. Be a verbal report that will eventually be followed by an official written report
D. Focus on the positive findings of the team

9.
The advantages of a Joint Commission on Accreditation of Heathcare Organizations (JCAHO) survey include all of the following EXCEPT:
A. JCAHO accreditation may favorably impact the state survey process.
B. Facilities that are accredited may be used as training sites for healthcare professionals.
C. Facilities that are accredited may be eligible for additional grants and other

funding.
D. The JCAHO survey is free to member organizations.

10.
The MOST IMPORTANT role of the nurse in the state survey process is:
A. Maintaining thorough, accurate documentation
B. Being familiar with federal and state regulations governing the operation of nursing homes
C. Being familiar with theJCAHO standards
D. Answering survey team members' questions

Chapter Fourteen

1.
A nurse was asked to join with peers to look at residents' charts to determine whether a recently implemented skin protocol had decreased the incidence or severity of pressure ulcers. The nurse was being asked to participate in a/an
A. Prospective audit
B. Concurrent audit
C. Retrospective audit
D. Outcome evalutation audit

2.
As compared to quality assurance, continuous quality improvement (CQI)
A. Is less comprehensive
B. Is concerned with clinical outcomes, cost, and customer satisfaction
C. Looks at how well employees do their job
D. Looks at care before it is given

3.
A staff nurse was explaining standards to a newly employed geriatric nursing assistant (GNA). The BEST explanation of standards is that they
A. Are the indicators of excellence
B. Provide caregivers with measures to use for comparison
C. Are nationally recognized hallmarks of good care
D. Provide survey teams with a fair, unbiased tool to measure facilities

4.
Structure standards are concerned with issues such as:
A. What care and how that care is given to residents
B. Whether grounds maintenance equipment is safe
C. Whether the care a resident receives accomplishes what is intended
D. What amount of time is acceptable for accomplishing a resident's admission assessment

5.
A director of nursing (DON) was reviewing residents' incident reports and noted a sudden increase in reported burn injuries. While talking to the kitchen staff, the DON learned that the kitchen had run out of lids and that the purchasing department had found some old lids. The old lids were slightly tighter on the cups. The DON called the purchasing department, and the lids were removed from the nursing units. The DON was serving what function?

A. Utilization review
B. Quality assessment
C. Risk management
D. Performance management

Chapter Fifteen

1.
In a professional negligence lawsuit, the plaintiff must prove:
A. A duty was owed and injury occurred
B. A duty was owed that was breached and caused injury to the patient
C. A duty was owed and the health care provider breached the duty
D. A duty was owed and monetary damages occurred

2.
During a professional negligence lawsuit, the nurse defendant tries to establish that he or she acted in the appropriate professional manner. Such a defense is called:
A. Customary institutional practice standard
B. Peer standard
C. Expert witness testimony
D. Ordinary prudent nurse standard

3.
One of the most significant steps nurses can take to prevent malpractice claims is to:
A. Carry malpractice insurance
B. Work at improving their own practices
C. Check with their supervisors before initiating any action
D. Avoid caring for suit-prone clients

4.
A nurse is convinced that the elders in her care do not want aggressive resuscitation measures. From an ethical decision-making point of view, such a belief is a/an
A. Environmental factor
B. Task factor
C. Nurse factor
D. Ethical factor

5.
A staff nurse questions the rightness of permitting a patient with potentially life-threatening respiratory problems to remain in the long term care facility where equipment such as a ventilator is not available. The concern is based on which type of factor affecting ethical decision making?
A. Task factor

B. Environmental factor
C. Nurse factor
D. Practice factor

6.
A nurse overhears a geriatric nursing assistant (GNA) say to a confused wandering patient "If you don't stop wandering, I'll have to see if you can be kept in your room." When questioned further, the GNA expresses grave concern that the patient is at risk for harm, having been found in the patient lounge trying to poke a pencil into a light socket. The facility promotes free movement of its patients. What is the BEST response for the nurse to make?
A. "I understand that you are concerned for the patient's safety, but we cannot restrict movement."
B. "You cannot threaten a patient."
C. "Just be sure to keep an eye out for the patient. I know how frustrating it can be."
D. "We will take the matter to the patient care advisory committee and ask how best to
keep the patient safe."

7.
A nurse goes to an inservice program on providing careful and complete complicated wound care for clients with stage IV pressure ulcers. The nurse is following which of the following standards of behavior from the ANA *Code for Nurses*?
A. The nurse participates in the profession's efforts to implement and improve standards of nursing.
B. The nurse maintains competence in nursing.
C. The nurse assumes responsibility and accountability for individual nursing judgment.
D. The nurse safeguards the client's right to privacy.

8.
When a nurse suspects that a nursing peer is practicing under the influence of alcohol, the observing nurse should:
A. Confront the individual personally
B. Talk with the immediate supervisor in an informal way
C. Ask to transfer to another unit to avoid legal liability
D. Record specific dates and behaviors observed

9.
Which of the following ANA *Code for Nurses* statements directly relates to the ethical issues involved in a nurse's administration of placebos?

A. The nurse provides services with respect for human dignity.
B. The nurse maintains competence in nursing.
C. The nurse assumes responsibility for individual nursing judgment and actions.
D. The nurse acts to safeguard the client from unethical, incompetent, or illegal practice.

10.
The nurse had a fragile man in his 80s as a client. When his heart stopped, he was resuscitated and awakened with tubes and machines. He begged to be allowed to die but was repeatedly resuscitated at the insistence of his wife and daughter. What document could have helped this man to obtain the dignified death he wanted?
A. Do not resuscitate order
B. Durable power of attorney for health care held by his daughter
C. Living will
D. No documents are currently available to cover this situation

TEST BANK ANSWERS

Each test bank item is classified by question number and by the chapter objective to which the question refers. For example, the first item covering chapter one, objective one is identified as **1(1)** under the heading **Chapter 1**. The rationale for each correct answer is presented. Finally, each item is described in terms of the step in the nursing process, the category of human need, and the cognitive level, which permits instructors to select items using NCLEX standard descriptors. For this test bank, the steps in the nursing process are identified as **assess, analysis, plan, implement, and evaluate.** The categories of human need are identified as safe, effective care environment **(SEC)**, physiological integrity **(physio)**, psychosocial integrity **(P/S)**, and health promotion and maintenance **(HP/M)**.

Chapter 1

1(1)
D
Elders 85 years and older typically have multiple health problems. Age 96 classifies as old old.
analysis, P/S, comprehension

2(1)
B
While only 5 percent of people over age 65 live in nursing homes, 30 percent to 40 percent of people over 65 can expect at least one admission to a nursing home.
assess, HP/M, knowledge

3(1)
C
Only 5 percent of people over age 65 live in nursing homes.
assess, HP/M, knowledge

4(2)
A
Social nutrition programs initiated by the Older Americans' Act of 1965 documented that improved nutrition prevents illness in elders.
analysis, HP/M, comprehension

5(2)
D

While gender, attitude toward aging, and fear of the health care system may affect health status, the major predictor is socioeconomic status. In general, the lower the socioeconomic status, the poorer the health status regardless of other factors.
> **analysis, physio, knowledge**

6(2)
C
Elders who are suspicious of the health care system demonstrate behaviors listed in A, B, and D. Elders who trust the health care system may well view their provider as "Godlike."
> **assess, P/S, comprehension**

7(3)
B
Because Mr. Jones is not physically impaired, he is able to meet his activities of daily living and because he has able adult supervision in the home, adult day care is the most appropriate health care setting.
> **plan, HP/M, comprehension**

8(3)
D
The nursing home is the appropriate setting for an elder who needs rehabilitation services and has no one at home who is able to provide care. A home health aide is able to provide care for a limited period each day.
> **plan, HP/M, comprehension**

Chapter 2

1(1)
C
Social security legislation was passed in the 1930s. Medicare legislation was passed in 1965. The Omnibus Budget Reconciliation Act was passed in the 1980s.
> **assess, SEC, knowledge**

2(1)
A
Medicare legislation was passed in 1965.
> **assess, SEC, knowledge**

3(1)
D

Because Mrs. Smith is independent and physically active, a life-care community would best meet her needs.
plan, P/S, comprehension

4(2)
B
With a history of trauma and chronic motor impairments, a head injury unit might best meet Mr. Higgins's needs and put him with others closer to his own age.
plan, SEC, comprehension

5(2)
A
A home health aide, if Mrs. Slaughter can afford one, would be the best choice.
plan, SEC, comprehension

6(2)
D
White women have the longest life expectancy of any cultural or ethnic group.
assess, physio, knowledge

7(2)
A
Short-stay residents typically are under age 75, have had an acute health problem, and are cognitively intact.
analysis, HP/M, knowledge

8(3)
D
The average length of stay for a nursing home resident admitted for living arrangements is approximately 2.5 years.
plan, HP/M, knowledge

9(3)
B
Severe, debilitating diseases are now being managed more successfully prolonging life, but creating a tremendous care burden. Congestive heart failure, stroke, and hip fracture are seen more commonly in the older adult.
assess, HP/M, knowledge

10(4)
C
Relocation syndrome should always be considered when a newly admitted resident has increased anxiety, hallucinations, or other cognitive difficulties. Delusional thinking is a description, not a cause of cognitive impairment. Over-hydration and sensory deprivation are possible causes for cognitive impairment but unlikely in so short a period.
  analysis, physio, comprehension

11(4)
B
Information helps clients to feel more in control and decreases anxiety. Information makes a threatening situation more understandable.
  implement, HP/M, application

12(5)
C
Medicare will pay up to 100 days after a qualifying 3-day stay in a hospital.
  plan, HP/M, knowledge

13
A
While B, C, and D are usually part of the survey process, resident outcomes is noted as the primary concern of the survey.
  assess, SEC, knowledge

14
D
The Joint Commission on Accreditation of Healthcare Organizations is the primary voluntary accrediting agency for health care agencies.
  assess, SEC, knowledge

Chapter 3

1(1)
D
Because Mr. Bishop has expressed concern over a normal age-related finding, it would be most important for the nurse to explain aging changes to the heart. Documentation and reporting are important, but not a priority. Checking resting heart rate is important as part of the physical but does not address his concern.
  implement, HP/M, application

2(1)

C
The nurse should know that Mrs. Steary may be experiencing orthostatic hypotension from age-related peripheral vascular inelasticity.
assess, physio, comprehension

3(1)
B
Lung compliance and intercostal muscle inelasticity decrease arterial oxygen levels. Prolonged activity requires increased oxygen. Heart rate usually does not increase but is not lower. Rapid walking is possible, and renal changes do not increase need for sodium replacement.
assess, physio, comprehension

4(1)
A
Dehydration, as evidenced by dry skin with poor turgor, in combination with decreased ciliary action causes secretions to thicken and remain in air passages. Coughing promotes clearing of the air passages. A respiratory rate of 20/min is normal. A weight gain of 0.5 pounds in 3 weeks is not clinically significant by itself.
analysis, SEC, application

5(1)
B
Elders usually need more time to learn material. Short sessions, with practice time, facilitates the learning process best.
plan, HP/M, application

6(1)
D
Loss of REM sleep, a normal age-related change, frequently causes elders to feel less rested.
implement, HP/M, comprehension

7(1)
D
Osteoporosis is irreversible. Men with higher testosterone levels tend to build bone. Osteoporosis may cause compression fractures of the spine and hip fractures. African-American women, as compared with women of other races, have more bone stock and usually do not experience severe osteoporosis.
implement, HP/M, comprehension

8(1)
B
Mrs. Garcia seems to have enough clothing and bedding. The room temperature is appropriate for most adults. However, the loss of subcutaneous tissue puts her at risk for excessive loss of body heat in what appears to be normal temperatures.
      analysis, physio, comprehension

9(1)
C
Benign prostatic hypertrophy can cause overflow incontinence, or "dribbling."
      analysis, physio, comprehension

10(2)
B
Androgen stimulates the bone marrow to produce red blood cells. Androgen production usually diminishes in men over age 80.
      analysis, physio, comprehension

11(2)
C
Elderly people have immune systems that are less effective because they have fewer white blood cells and fewer lymphocytes.
      analysis, physio, application

12(2)
A
Decreased thyroid hormones are responsible for hypothyroidism, which is common in elderly woman.
      analysis, physio, application

13(2)
B
An elevated BUN level is not uncommon in the elderly population. A better measure of kidney function is the serum creatinine concentration.
      analysis, physio, comprehension

14(2)
D
Serum creatinine concentration is the most accurate indicator of kidney function. A low serum creatinine concentration means the kidneys are less able to excrete drugs and may require that dosages be lowered to prevent toxic build-up.
      analysis, SEC, application

15(3)
A
Retirement may be stressful and perceived as a loss. Depression may result. Iron deficiency anemia and immune system dysfunction generally do not make life senseless. Mr. Rosenburg is not demonstrating delusional thinking.
        analysis, P/S, application

16(3)
C
Church may serve a social function, but few view it as solely social. Religion and church are viewed as very helpful in stressful times, and there is a strong association between religion and well-being.
        assess, P/S, knowledge

17(3)
C
A, B, and D offer false reassurance. C opens the interview and permits the resident to express her feelings and fears in a therapeutic communication.
        implement, P/S, application

18(4)
B
The PASSARR documents screening specifically for mental illness or mental retardation.
        assess, P/S, knowledge

19(4)
A
The LPN/LVN is responsible for gathering data for the initial assessment according to agency policy. The accuracy and completion of the nursing assessment data base is the responsibility of the RN.
        implement, SEC, comprehension

20(4)
D
The minimum data set (MDS) and resident assessment protocols (RAPs) is an interdisciplinary assessment tool that serves as the basis for interdisciplinary resident care planning.
        assess, SEC, knowledge

21(4)
C
Assessment of residents in a nursing home differs from the shift-to-shift assessments of patients in acute care settings in that physical assessments on all residents may not be done by the nurse every day.
assess, SEC, comprehension

Chapter 4

1(1)
C
Neuropathy decreases sensation and proprioception, thus increasing the risk for falls. Diabetic neuropathy does not significantly add to the risk of confusion, bunions, or deep venous thrombosis.
analysis, physio, application

2(1)
B
Parkinson's disease leaves residents stiff and also affects balance. Hand tremors and mental status generally do not increase fall risk for residents with Parkinson's disease. Use of a walker diminishes fall risk.
analysis, physio, application

3(1)
D
A, B, and C are normal age-related changes and do not directly increase risk for falls. Impaired vision, especially cataracts, increases fall risk.
analysis, SEC, comprehension

4(1)
D
A and C involve changes to sensation that increase fall risk. B causes increased urinary frequency and nocturia, which also increases fall risk. D is a skin disorder that is not directly associated with fall risk.
analysis, SEC, application

5(1)
A
B and D follow proper safety and body mechanic standards. The multilevel cart is large enough for easy viewing and in a location where both staff and residents might expect it. A pencil on the floor is an unexpected, difficult to observe, slippery item that sharply escalates fall risk.
evaluate, SEC, application

6(1)
C
Knowing the time and location of falls permits using A, B, and D in context to plan appropriate interventions. Without C, the other data is unrelated to falls.
analysis, SEC, application

7(1)
B
A, C, and D are recommended safety interventions that decrease falls. Toileting frequently will decrease falls, but a 6-to 8-hour regimen is too long for elders who may have weakened bladder muscles.
implement, SEC, comprehension

8(2)
D
Although fall trauma rarely causes breathing difficulty, it is important to determine that the fall was not the result of respiratory or cardiac arrest.
implement, SEC, application

9(2)
B
Other than head injury, fractures of the hip are the largest concern following a resident fall.
analysis, SEC, comprehension

10(2)
B
A hip fracture in the elderly may not demonstrate all the classic symptoms. Mrs. Tranh's physician may want a thorough evaluation including x-rays. Documentation, communication, and monitoring are appropriate only if fractures or other trauma is completely ruled out.
analysis, physio, comprehension

11(3)
A
B and C are normal age-related changes and do not directly increase risk for pressure ulcers. An unsteady gait increases fall risk but not the risk for pressure ulcers. Undernutrition, with loss of subcutaneous tissue, substantially increases the risk for pressure ulcers.
analysis, SEC, comprehension

12(3)
C

Haloperidol (Haldol) is given to decrease hallucinations, both visual and auditory. Haloperidol has no direct effect on continence. The drug may act as a chemical restraint and increase immobility, which can cause pressure ulcers.
> **evaluate, SEC, application**

13(3)
C
The Braden Scale is scored from low to high, with the lowest scores identifying the greatest risk. A score of six is the lowest score possible.
> **analysis, physio, comprehension**

14(4)
A
Stage I pressure ulcers are reddened and do not blanche with finger pressure. The skin remains reddened. Stages II through IV involve open skin.
> **analysis, physio, comprehension**

15(4)
D
African-Americans usually have darker skin, making assessment for blanching or prolonged reddening more difficult than among lighter-skinned individuals. Age, diagnosis, and location are facts that increase the risk but do not alter the assessment
> **assess, physio, comprehension**

16(4)
B
Eschar makes assessment for staging pressure ulcers more difficult because it is impossible to determine the depth of the ulcer until the eschar is removed. Drainage, immobility, incontinence, and poor nutrition are risk factors for pressure ulcers.
> **assess, physio, comprehension**

17(4)
C
A Stage III ulcer that has purulent drainage indicates infection. A yellow wound is usual with an infection. A reddened, swollen wound indicates tissue damage within the first 72 hours. A black wound indicates nonhealing and eschar, information not given in the stem.
> **analysis, physio, comprehension**

18(4)
C
A Stage III ulcer that has purulent drainage indicates infection. A yellow wound is usual with an infection. A reddened, swollen wound indicates tissue damage within the first 72 hours. A black wound indicates nonhealing and eschar, information not given in the stem.
analysis, physio, comprehension

19(5)
B
The resident demonstrates the classic profile for stress incontinence: older age, multiparity, history of abdominal surgeries, and symptoms with increased abdominal pressure.
analysis, physio, comprehension

20(5)
D
Fecal impaction may cause incontinence. A increases the possibility of bladder infection. Toileting every 6 to 8 hours is too infrequent for most elders. Eating soft, cooked foods may increase constipation.
plan, physio, comprehension

21(5)
A
Stress incontinence may be helped by muscle strengthening exercises in the pelvic floor. Interventions B, C, and D are useful strategies for overflow incontinence.
plan, physio, comprehension

22(5)
C
Interventions A and B are useful with stress incontinence. Intervention D is useful with overflow incontinence. Frequent toileting is useful with functional incontinence.
plan, physio, comprehension

23(6)
D
Acute delirium may be caused by A, B, and/or C. Adequate hydration should help rather than add to the cognitive problem.
analysis, physio, comprehension

24(6)
C

Loss of interest in activities, sleep difficulties, poor appetite, and poor concentration are evidence of depression.

analysis, P/S, comprehension

25(6)
A

The cognitive impairments are typical of dementia. Mr. Ewing's age, gender, and medical condition make multi-infarct dementia the most likely diagnosis.

analysis, P/S, comprehension

26(7)
B

Avoiding triggers that aggravate behaviors is an appropriate intervention. Frequent changes of routine or a noisy, perplexing environment may cause increased confusion for the resident.

plan, SEC, knowledge

27(7)
D

A, B, and C are strategies for working with paranoid or hallucinating residents. Placing a large NO sign or plastic tape across doorways is generally an effective method to discourage wanderers from entering rooms.

implement, SEC, comprehension

28(7)
A

B, C, and D are strategies for wanderers. A quiet non-stimulating, routine environment decreases screaming.

implement, SEC, comprehension

29(7)
C

A, B, and D are devices that do not restrict mobility but remind residents that they need assistance to get out of chairs.

implement, SEC, comprehension

30(8)
B

A weight loss of 3 pounds over 5 weeks is not out of range. The body mass index range is 20 to 25. A low serum albumin concentration is a good, but late indicator. The thyroxine PAB is the best early test of malnutrition.

analysis, SEC, comprehension

31(8)
B
The nurse must determine whether the weight gain is actual or the result of an error in obtaining the weight. The next step is to determine whether the weight loss is from fluid loss or actual malnutrition. Notification of physician and follow-up weights are appropriate later steps.
    implement, SEC, application

32(8)
D
A low serum albumin concentration, low cholesterol level, low white blood cell count, and poor wound healing all point to malnutrition.
    analysis, physio, application

33(9)
C
A verbal and written advance directive from a resident should be followed. D is correct but does not address the right of the resident to predetermine his medical therapy choice.
    implement, SEC, comprehension

34(9)
D
A gastrostomy tube or jejunostomy tube have the lowest risk of aspiration.
    analysis, SEC, knowledge

35(9)
A
For a first-time percutaneous endoscopic gastrostomy tube feeding, x-ray confirmation of tube placement is the first safety check. Checking to sure the tube is still in the correct place should be done next.
    implement, SEC, comprehension

36(9)
C
A, B, and D are common complications of tube feedings. Feeding tubes do not impair mobility.
    evaluate, SEC, knowledge

37(10)
B
Recording the bowel movements does not prevent constipation unless something is done with the information. Limiting visitors is unnecessary. Disimpacting a bowel is not a preventive intervention but a restorative intervention. Establishing a bowel routine is a preventive strategy for constipation.
        plan, physio, comprehension

38(10)
C
Assessment is the first step of the nursing process, and with abdominal assessment, auscultation precedes palpation. A review of food consumption might be useful for preventive information but will not address the distention and discomfort.
        implement, physio, comprehension

39(10)
B
Antibiotic therapy may diminish the normal intestinal bacteria and permit pathogenic bacteria such as *Clostridium difficile* to flourish. Her water and food consumption are normal. Eating in a dining room is not a cause for diarrhea.
        analysis, physio, comprehension

40(10)
D
Fluid administration to prevent dehydration is the most important intervention. A, B, and C may be appropriate depending upon the cause of the diarrhea.
        implement, physio, comprehension

Chapter 5

1(1)
B
Polypharmacy is common among elders. Using one source for medications aids pharmacists to check for drug interactions and duplication.
        analysis, SEC, comprehension

2(1)
D
Elders at high risk have numerous chronic illnesses, tend to self-medicate, have health care providers who do not know drugs well, and who prescribe drugs to counter side effects of other drugs.
analysis, SEC, comprehension

3(1)
B
Knowledge of drugs, lower doses for the elderly, and frequent review for appropriateness lower the incidence of polypharmacy.
evaluate, SEC, comprehension

4(2)
C
Insulin is injected, not absorbed, through the gut. Insulin has no discernable impact on peptic ulcer disease. Insulin requirements are adjusted to the activity of the resident. Poor subcutaneous tissue deposits may prevent proper administration of the insulin.
analysis, SEC, application

5(2)
D
Verapamil and furosemide are protein-bound for distribution. The low serum albumin decreases the distribution of these drugs. Other test values are within normal range.
analysis, SEC, application

6(2)
A
Mr. Stanka's history of alcohol use should alert the nurse to impaired drug metabolism. B, C, and D are observations that might be appropriate for any resident with the stated diagnoses.
evaluate, SEC, application

7(3)
B
The lowest dose of a medication should be tried before increasing the dose. Increases should be done gradually.
plan, SEC, comprehension

8(3)
D

Bleeding gums is a common adverse effect of nonsteroidal anti-inflammatory drugs. Drowsiness, dry mouth, and orthostatic hypotension are common with other classes of medication.

evaluate, SEC, application

9(4)
D

Nurses frequently express concern that elders are more at risk for sedation and respiratory depression. A, B, and C are evidence of appropriate pain control.

plan, SEC, comprehension

10(4)
C

A, B, and D are common inaccurate beliefs elders frequently have about pain and pain management. Residents need frequent reassurance that they are not a bother or a complainer.

plan, HP/M, comprehension

11(4)
C

A, B, and D are evidence of acute pain. Mr. Schwartz meets the profile for chronic pain.

assess, physio, comprehension

12(4)
B

A and C may require the resident to respond at a higher level than they are capable. Interviewing the physician does not assess the resident's pain. Observation of pain behaviors may be the most accurate indicator of a resident's pain.

assess, physio, comprehension

13(4)
D

Giving acetaminophen would violate the written order. B and C might be effective for mild to moderate pain but are very likely ineffective for severe pain. Calling the physician and reporting the resident's level of pain advocates for the resident.

implement, SEC, application

14(5)
C
C is hypertonic and the rate may put this elder at risk for fluid overload. A, B, and D are isotonic solutions and the rate is appropriate for the resident's age and medical diagnoses.
analysis, SEC, application

15(5)
A
Infection is the major complication with partial parenteral nutrition and total parenteral nutrition. B, and C indicate problems usually associated with events other than parenteral nutrition. D may be a expected outcome given the resident's medical diagnosis.
evaluate, SEC, application

Chapter 6

1(1)
C
Crowded living space and visitors increase the risk of acute infections. A and B are at the low end of normal intake, and D is the recommended prophylaxis to prevent an acute respiratory infection.
assess, HP/T, comprehension

2(1)
A
Of all the infection control strategies available, conscientious handwashing is the most important for prevention of infection. B, C, and D are appropriate strategies but secondary to handwashing.
plan, HP/T, application

3(1)
B
The resident is at high risk for a urinary tract infection. A and D are appropriate interventions for residents at high risk or having respiratory infections. C does not indicate an infectious process.
plan, HP/T, application

4(2)
C
Increased temperature is frequent with dehydration. A, B, and D are seen with fluid overload.
assess, physio, comprehension

5(2)
D
Crackles in the lung bases indicate excess fluid leaking into alveolar spaces. A, B, and C are indicators of fluid volume deficit.
        assess, physio, comprehension

6(2)
B
Oral replacement therapy is the treatment of choice for fluid volume deficit in elderly residents. A, C, and D are therapies for fluid overload
        plan, physio, comprehension

7(2)
A
Residents are frequently dyspneic with fluid overload and need oxygen support. B, C, and D are interventions for fluid volume deficit.
        plan, physio, comprehension

8(3)
D
The symptoms and history are consistent with a potassium deficit. A, B, and C do not match the history and symptoms.
        assess, physio, comprehension

9(3)
B
Non–potassium-sparing diuretics are the most common cause of potassium deficits. A, C, and D have little or no impact on potassium balance.
        analysis, SEC, application

10(3)
B
The symptoms and history are consistent with a sodium deficit. A, C, and D do not match the history and symptoms.
        assess, physio, comprehension

11(4)
B
Mrs. Polevoy has the classic symptoms of diabetic ketoacidosis. A, C, and D do not match the symptoms or history.
        analysis, physio, application

12(4)
D
Mr. Siemonds has the classic symptoms of hyperglycemic, hyperosmolar, and nonketotic coma. The nurse should expect a blood sugar greater than 600 mg/dL.
    analysis, physio, comprehension

13(5)
B
The resident's history suggests the possibility of an atypical myocardial infarction (MI). A might be a possible factor, but the continued pain unrelieved suggests an MI. C and D do not match the history.
    analysis, physio, application

14(5)
B
Nitroglycerin is given sublingually for angina for a maximum of three tablets 5 minutes apart. The resident should be put at complete rest if angina or an MI is suspected. Oxygen is usually not started for angina.
    plan, physio, comprehension

15(6)
C
The skin over the affected area is swollen and warm. A, B, and D are symptoms of acute arterial occlusion.
    analysis, physio, comprehension

16(6)
A
A is characteristic of acute arterial occlusion. B, C, and D are customary with deep venous thrombosis.
    analysis, physio, comprehension

Chapter 7

1(1)
C
Clinical pathways are more beneficial for short-stay residents. A, B, and D are long-term residents.
    plan, SEC, application

2(1)
B
A record of nonachievement of outcomes for a clinical pathway is called a variance report.
   implement, SEC, comprehension

3(2)
A
B, C, and D are documentation errors that the nurse should avoid.
   implement, SEC, knowledge

4(2)
C
A, B, and D are all reasons why a nurse documents a resident's progress.
   analysis, SEC, comprehension

5(3)
A
Documentation that follows a timeline and describes events in chronological order is traditional narrative charting. B and C are alternative charting methods. D does not appear on the resident's comprehensive medical record.
   analysis, SEC, comprehension

6(3)
C
A is an advantage of PIE charting. B and D are disadvantages of narrative charting.
   analysis, SEC, knowledge

7(4)
B
The treatment, because it contained antibiotic therapy, will need to be recorded on the medication administration record. A and C are not appropriate because the problem is known and being actively treated. D is usually used to record daily activities and routine and ongoing treatments.
   implement, SEC, knowledge

8(4)
D
A, B, and C are actions that are legally inadvisable.
   analysis, SEC, knowledge

Chapter 8

1(1)
A
B, C, and D are incocrrect definitions.
   analysis, HP/T, knowledge

2(1)
C
A and B are important for health protection, but each is incomplete. D is an appropriate long-term goal for health promotion. C is the most comprehensive focus for this patient.
   plan, HP/T, application

3(2)
D
A ,B, and C are each opposite to current trends.
   analysis, HP/T, knowlege

4(2)
B
A and D are aimed specifically at the problems of confusion. D is aimed at a specific physiologic function that may prevent a problem.
   implement, HP/T, comprehension

5(3)
A
A teaching program should begin with an assessment of what the resident knows about his health problem(s). B and C are interventions, not assessments. D is planning, not assessment.
   assess, HP/T, application

6(3)
D
A, B, and C are important safety considerations but does not evaluate the resident's learning.
   evaluate, HP/T, comprehension

7(4)
C
Elders tend to be less confused early in the morning. A, B, and D are strategies that the nurse might consider but are less likely to be successful.
   plan, HP/T, comprehension

8(4)
B
A might distract the elder rather than help. C and D are contraindicated for best learning conditions.
plan, HP/T, comprehension

Chapter 9

1(1)
B
A is inappropriate because the patient requires intensive physical therapy, not acute care. C and D are inappropriate because the patient requires more care than these settings provide.
analysis, SEC, comprehension

2(1)
C
A offers false reassurance. B and D do not give the patient the information needed to for reassurance or an opportunity to further express her feelings.
evaluate, P/S, comprehension

3(2)
A
B and C are incorrect because both state and federal regulations must be met. D is incorrect because state surveys are mandatory.
analysis, SEC, knowledge

4(2)
B
A and C do not exist. D does not accredit subacute units.
assess, SEC, knowledge

5(3)
A
B and C do not offer seamless transfer or the substitute for continued hospital care. D does not provide the patient with the 24-hour care that is required.
analysis, SEC, comprehension

6(3)
C
A and B usually do not specialize in long-term problems, such as ventilator-dependent patients. Home with only daily visits does not provide a safe level of

management for the patient.
>**analysis, SEC, comprehension**

7(4)
D
A, B, and C, though good experience, does not prepare the nurse to care for ventilator- dependent residents.
>**analysis, SEC, comprehension**

8(4)
B
A is too little. C and D are too great. B is the usual formula for staffing.
>**analysis, SEC, knowlege**

9(5)
A
B is incorrect because the case manager may coordinate care across several health care settings. C is incorrect because the number of identified outcomes has no defined limit. D is only partially correct because all resident outcomes might not maximize benefits to cost.
>**analysis, SEC, comprehension**

Chapter 10

1(1)
D
A, B, and C usually do not have stockholders who receive dividends on their investments in the company or facility.
>**analysis, SEC, comprehension**

2(1)
B
A is incorrect since all care needs may not be met by a single facility. C may not be possible. One hopes profits are used wisely, but there is no legal requirement for that to happen.
>**assess, SEC, comprehension**

3(2)
D
A, coming in under budget, is not the primary responsibility. B and C are incorrect because care must be given within budgeted costs.
      evaluate, SEC, comprehension

4(2)
B
A, C, and D are responsible for some of the nursing home activities, but the nursing home administrator (NHA) is accountable to the board of NHA for his or her practice.
      assess, SEC, knowledge

5(3)
A
Questions regarding newly ordered drugs should always be clarified first with the ordering physician. The consultant pharmacist is the second best resource.
      plan, SEC, knowledge

6(3)
D
Assessment is the first step to developing an adequate plan of care. Weight loss may occur for a variety of reasons, one of which is inadequate calorie intake. A and B are appropriate after determining the amount the resident is routinely eating. C is appropriate if the resident is eating poorly because of mechanical factors.
      plan, SEC, comprehension

7(4)
C
A, B, and D are laundry, maintenance, and central office staff functions, respectively.
      analysis, SEC, knowledge

8(4)
D
A, B, and C are medical records consultant, staff development, and maintenance functions, respectively.
      implement, SEC, knowledge

9(5)
B
Speech-language pathologists are specifically educated to diagnose and treat

swallowing problems.
>**plan, SEC, comprehension**

Chapter 11

1(1)
B
Large equipment purchases are capital budget items.
>**analysis, SEC, comprehension**

2(1)
A
The director of nursing (DON) may occasionally provide direct care to clients, but administrative duties generally do not permit more than infrequent care opportunities.
>**analysis, SEC, comprehension**

3(2)
C
The requirements of the DON position have increased significantly, and many agencies are now requiring the DON to have a baccalaureate degree.
>**analysis, SEC, knowledge**

4(2)
D
The assistant director of nursing (ADON) is usually responsible for staffing and work schedules, although the ADON may do other delegated duties that the DON views as appropriate.
>**analysis, SEC, comprehension**

5(3)
A
Assessment of quality care permits planning to achieve the same or higher levels of quality. Evaluation tells where the care level is as a reflection of current efforts and programs for improvement.
>**analysis, SEC, application**

6(3)
D
The QI committee is an interdisciplinary committee that includes infection control, risk management, utilization review and clinical studies.

analysis, SEC, comprehension

7(3)
B
Risk management is specifically directed at improving safety and preventing medical malpractice.
assess, SEC, knowledge

8(4)
A
Task-oriented, specialized functions are the hallmarks of functional nursing.
analysis, SEC, comprehension

9(4)
D
The newest model for nursing care delivery is resident-centered care.
analysis, SEC, comprehension

10(5)
C
Geriatric nursing assistants (GNAs) provide direct care, such as bathing and mobility activities and bedmaking, for residents.
assess, SEC, knowledge

11(5)
B
Geriatric medical asssistants, after 1 year of experience as GNAs and an additional course of study, administer oral and certain topical medications.
assess, SEC, knowledge

12(6)
D
The case manager collaborates, monitors progress, and acts as resident advocate. While being financially responsible and aware, it is not the role of the case manager to impose budgetary constraints on resident care.
analysis, SEC, comprehension

Chapter 12

1(1)
C
The charge nurse is part responsible for the atmosphere on the unit. Encouraging

residents to participate on the residents' council helps to give them a voice in their surroundings.

analysis, P/S, comprehension

2(1)
B
The role of the charge nurse is being responsible for nursing staff for a period of time. The charge nurse is not always an RN, nor is it a full-time management position.

analysis, SEC, knowledge

3(2)
C
In many nursing homes, the GNAs get a report on their residents from the charge nurse. A complete shift report is detailed and includes medical and nursing objectives for each resident.

plan, SEC, comprehension

4(2)
B
Personal comments and unprofessional observations should not be a part of a shift report.

implement, SEC, comprehension

5(3)
C
The nurse is responsible for ensuring that the nursing assistant has the knowledge, skills, and ability to carry out the assignment. In addition, the nurse is responsible for supervising the nursing assistant to ensure that the task is carried out correctly.

analysis, SEC, comprehension

6(3)
D
When making nursing care assignments, the charge nurse must consider the staff, their knowledge, the needs of the client, and continuity of care. Cost per staff hour of care is an important management concern, but not for nursing care assignments.

analysis, SEC, comprehension

7(3)
A common reason for underdelegation is perfectionism and the perceived loss of control by the nurse.

analysis, SEC, comprehension

8(3)
C
Delegation to get rid of an unpleasant job task is an inappropriate reason to delegate. Job enrichment, better time utilization, and best use of personnel are all good reasons to delegate a nursing care task.
analysis, SEC, application

9(3)
D
A, B, and C are elements in good delegation. The nurse is required to direct an supervise as deemed appropriate. Even if the staff member does not request supervision, the nurse is still accountable for the supersion.
analysis, SEC, application

10(3)
C
A, B, and D are essential for good delegation. The staff member is not given full discretion on delegated functions.
analysis, SEC, application

11(4)
C
Open discussion in an atmosphere of trust and commitment are the foundations for collaboration.
implement, SEC, application

12(4)
D
All units will lose some of what they need with Mrs. Grantham's proposal. Staff will feel—and correctly so—that they had to give up something that they needed.
analysis, SEC, comprehension

13(4)
B
By not confronting the rude behavior, the individual has chosen to avoid a conflict.
analysis, SEC, comprehension

14(5)
A
Shared decision making, delegation, participation, and feedback reflect a democratic approach.

analysis, SEC, comprehension

15(5)
D
The characteristics describe the autocratic style of leadership.
analysis, SEC, comprehension

Chapter 13

1(1)
A
The survey is an inspection to determine compliance with state and federal laws. The survey is unannounced and nonvoluntary
analysis, SEC, knowledge

2(2)
B
Survey findings are a matter of public record and must be accessible to anyone who wishes to review them.
analysis, SEC, knowledge

3(2)
C
Environmental quality assessments observe how the physical surroundings affect residents' well-being.
analysis, SEC, comprehension

4(3)
A
Both the resident and family councils are official groups that meet regularly to discuss care issues and the operation of the facility as it affects the residents.
assess, SEC, knowledge

5(3)
B
The family council is the appropriate body to which Mrs. Smith should take her concerns, because she is not a resident of the facility.
plan, SEC, comprehension

6(4)
C
Only in very unusual circumstances would a drug therapy review surveyor look

133

at the diet sheet. The physicians' orders sheet, medication administration record (MAR), and laboratory studies are the common documents used.
  analysis, SEC, knowledge

7(4)
D
The physician must clearly identify the purpose of the medications ordered. Common places to note this are the order sheet, progress note, and, by transcription, the MAR.
  plan, SEC, knowledge

8(5)
B
The survey team will give the facility administrator a written report of the deficiencies found during the survey. The focus of the exit conference is to identify deficiencies.
  plan, SEC, knowledge

9(6)
D
The Joint Commission on Accreditation of Healthcare Organizations survey, though voluntary, is paid for by the requesting facility.
  analysis, SEC, knowledge

10(7)
B
The most important role of the nurse is to be knowledgeable about the federal and state regulations governing long term care.
  analysis, SEC, comprehension

Chapter 14

1(1)
B
The nurse was being asked to participate in a concurrent audit while the residents were receiving care.
  assess, SEC, knowledge

2(1)
B
Continuous quality improvement (CQI) is a broad-based program to look at all aspects of life in the facility, with the intent of making constant improvements.
  analysis, SEC, knowledge

3(2)
A
Standards define quality or excellence.
      analysis, SEC, knowledge

4(2)
B
Structure standards are concerned with the physical plant, equipment, financial resources, and policies.
      analysis, SEC, comprehension

5(3)
C
Risk management focuses on the monitoring and prevention of accidents, incidents, and malpractice.
      analysis, SEC, comprehension

Chapter 15

1(1)
B
The four elements of professional negligence are duty, breach of duty, injury, and causality, or that the breach of duty was the cause of injury.
      analysis, SEC, knowledge

2(1)
D
The defendant in a professional negligence lawsuit attempts to establish that the care rendered met the ordinary prudent nurse standard of care.
      analysis, SEC, knowledge

3(1)
B
Keeping up to date and increasing skills and knowledge are the most effective ways to prevent malpractice claims.
      plan, SEC, comprehension

4(2)
C
Beliefs occur within the nurse and are thus nurse factors.
      analysis, SEC, comprehension

5(2)

B
Availabilty of appropriate technology is an environmental factor.
analysis, SEC, comprehension

6(3)
D
The nurse identifies the conflict between freedom of movement and responsibility for safety. The patient care advisory committee is the institutional sounding board for these dilemmas.
implement, SEC, application

7(3)
B
The ongoing acquisition of nursing knowledge to improve nursing care is the foundation for maintaining competence in nursing.
analysis, SEC, comprehension

8(4)
D
Because the alcohol consumption is not confirmed, the nurse should record observations and dates. The observing nurse is required to intervene directly if, in professional opinion, the peer nurse is unsafe to provide care to patients.
implement, SEC, application

9(4)
D
Administering placebos is unethical because a deliberate falsehood is involved. The falsehood violates the patient's personhood and autonomy.
analysis, SEC, application

10(4)
C
A living will can spell out the wishes of the terminally ill. Consent of the family is sought but not required.
analysis, SEC, comprehension